Metabolic Living

TABLE OF CONTENTS

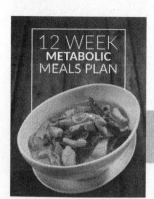

PAGE 113

INTRODUCTION

Hello, and welcome to *Metabolic Renewal*. I could not be more excited that you are embarking on this revolutionary program designed specifically to help women tap into the unique attributes of their female metabolisms, and to use that as an *advantage* to lose weight, look great and thrive.

This program is like no other on the market. It is the culmination of 25+ years of working in the trenches as a personal trainer, across the desk as a physician, and as a life coach and counselor for women all ages and in all stages of life.

Metabolic Renewal is the first hormone-focused body change program ever developed specifically for women. It is also architected to be the last diet and exercise program you will ever need. That's because it gives you the tools and knowledge needed to personalize the program so you can adapt how you eat, exercise and live in response to how your body's natural cycles, rhythms and hormones change as you age.

If you don't know me, let me introduce myself. My name is Dr. Jade Teta. I know, it is a strange name. My mom, who is also my best friend, loved the name Jade and when she found out she was pregnant with me she decided that it was the going to be my name whether I turned out to be a boy or a girl. I am sure she had no idea I would turn out to be a big, burly, linebacker-looking dude, but I have learned to embrace the name nonetheless.

You might be wondering: How did a guy like me become such an expert in female metabolism? That is an interesting story.

I have been in the fitness industry for almost 30 years, and over 75% of my clients are women. As you know, women are a lot more proactive when it comes to health and fitness than men.

Women also learn from the time they begin menstruating that their hormones are directly related to the way look, function and feel. Typically, men don't figure that out until close to their fifth or sixth decade, when they begin to see their testosterone levels fall.

As a result of working with women, I was forced to learn all I could about female metabolism. I made it my business to learn everything there is to know about the unique attributes of female metabolism and its hormonal strengths and challenges. I've built my results and reputation on that knowledge.

In this program, you are finally going to get a program designed for women, and most importantly, a specific woman: You.

You are going to learn things you have never been told, and this understanding will forever change the way you think about dieting. For example, did you know that estrogen is a lot like the female version of testosterone? And that during certain times of the month when it is a little bit higher you can eat more, tolerate more stress, and your workout results will be intensified?

Did you know that progesterone is a hormone that helps stabilize mood, blocks the action of stress hormones like cortisol, and results in the body being less able to tolerate extreme diet and exercise approaches?

Did you know that at menopause the female metabolism becomes more reactive to certain types of foods and far more sensitive to stress? Because of this, the diet and exercise approaches that worked when you were younger will not work now. However, there are simple and powerful changes you can make to turn menopausal metabolism back on and begin restoring metabolic fat burning.

You might be wondering why you have never heard this information before. There is a good reason for that, and I am going to explain. But first you should understand that this is just the tip of the iceberg.

One of the most profound things you will learn about your female metabolism is how it has an advantage over men when it comes to one of the most powerful fat-burning, anti-aging hormones known. Human growth hormone (HGH), especially when combined with estrogen, is the female fat-loss secret. In this program, you are going to learn exactly how to harness this powerful hormonal cocktail.

Why don't you know this already?

I will be honest. Research on women as it pertains to health, fitness and weight loss is not easy to find. It may not be that surprising for you to learn that the vast majority of fitness research is done on young males. In fact, I am not aware of a single commercial exercise program that understands the unique hormonal strengths of being female, and how to leverage that.

Think about this for a minute. You have been following advice and doing programs built on research that was done on men, not women. Not only that, but these men were mostly college-aged. Not only is a young man light years different from a young woman, but he has almost nothing in common with a mature woman.

In fact, most of these programs are using information gleaned from studying twenty-year-old male bodybuilders. When women are addressed, it is young fit female athletes who represent a tiny sample of the women out there.

What about women who are new moms? What about high-level executive women under stress? How about women in their late thirties and early forties who are seeing their metabolism slow down?

What about women going through the tumultuous swings of perimenopause? How about the women who are actively in menopause or past menopause? How about women who have unique hormonal situations that men don't ever deal with, things like polycystic ovarian syndrome (PCOS), estrogen dominance, hypothyroid and others?

If you have felt like you are following all the so called "rules" and not getting any results, it is because you have been following the wrong rules for you.

All this male-dominated research and rhetoric is going to change in this program. I am going to teach you how to turn your natural female hormonal cycles into fuel that fires your fat-loss efforts.

And if you are menopausal, or have other metabolic challenges, like PCOS or estrogen dominance, I am going to teach you how and why they are slowing you down, and why going harder with exercise or more extreme with diet is the wrong approach.

You see, as a woman, you have hormonal strengths you are not aware of and are not exploiting. Notice how I said "hormonal strengths"? You are probably not used to thinking about female hormonal changes as a strength, but they are.

The hormone estrogen is the key. This hormone does everything testosterone does for men. It helps you sculpt lean tissue. It provides that beautiful hourglass shape. It buffers against stress-induced fat gains, and it even amplifies fat burning.

You have probably never heard estrogen talked about in this way, but it is true, and all of these effects are amplified by using one small hack into the female cycle. That hack is HGH.

HGH builds muscle and burns fat at the same time, something notoriously difficult to do. It also tightens connective tissue and may enhance the quality and look of your skin. This is why many researchers call it the "youth hormone."

As I alluded to, women produce more HGH than men during exercise. This is the empowering insight that has allowed me to get amazing results with countless women around the world.

But not just any type of exercise will do. Female-specific workouts that leverage your hormonal cycle and special techniques aimed at HGH production are needed to get the most out of this hormone.

That is what you will get in this program. This is female-targeted fat loss at its finest that will help you reach your full female metabolic potential.

You are also going to be given an upgraded understanding of your metabolism that will put the outdated articles on the Internet and those ancient diet books in your local bookstore to shame.

The real secret to understanding your metabolism is this: Diet and exercise are not the only thing you need to be aware of. In fact, as a woman, there are two other areas that are even more important.

Imagine your metabolism as a pyramid made of four sections. I call these four sections the 4Ms. The base is large and strong, with each section becoming narrower until you reach the pronounced peak at the top.

MINDSET

When it comes to your female metabolism, the strong base you need to be focusing on is not diet or exercise. The base is mindset or mindful living.

What you don't realize is that your metabolism, compared to a man's, is far more stress-sensitive. This makes sense, given that women are the childbearers. The female metabolism needs to be more in tune with its environment because in ancient times this is what allowed female intuition to know whether becoming pregnant would be a good idea or not.

This means that to achieve optimal health and tap into your full fat-burning potential, you need to learn how to reduce stress and live life in tune with the natural rhythms of your environment. In this program, you are going to learn how to master stress and turn it to your advantage.

MOVEMENT

The next section of the pyramid is movement. I am not talking about exercise here. You have been wrongly led to believe that movement and exercise are the same thing. They are not, and as a woman this is an especially important distinction.

Exercise research has told us that a component of metabolism called non-exercise associated thermogenesis (NEAT) makes up 15% of our changeable metabolism. Exercise is only 5%. And this is huge for your female metabolic expression.[1]

This why women who walk a lot remain so thin compared to women who don't, whether they exercise or not. As a woman, walking and other activities that are not exercise—gardening, walking, fidgeting, taking the stairs, etc.—sensitize the body to your hormonal system and reduce cortisol.

MEALS

The next two blocks on the pyramid are meals (what you eat) and metabolics (how you exercise.) These are powerful movers of your body if and only if you get the mindfulness and movement pieces correct. Once the lower bases of the pyramid are solid, a sustainable diet and smart exercise program can turn on the most stubborn female metabolism.

The diet you will follow will be unlike anything you have ever seen. This is because rather than making you follow a restrictive diet that eliminates entire food groups, you will instead focus on finding the foods that work for you. You are unique metabolically, psychologically and in your personal preferences.

This dietary approach teaches you how to be a metabolic detective rather than a dieter. You will learn a cyclical eating approach that flows with the wisdom of your natural hormone cycle and rhythms and works with your exercise efforts. In the end, you will create a diet built for you, by you.

METABOLICS (EXERCISE)

Finally, there are the metabolics, or exercise. The workouts in this program are designed to turn on every advantage you have as a female. The most striking aspect is the "smarter, not harder" approach. In just 15 minutes, only three times a week, you will amplify your metabolic output so you are burning fat and tightening your body even on the days you are not working out.

The exercises are engineered and sequenced in specific ways to create a simultaneous breathless and burning response. It's these exercises that amplify HGH production and produce the body you want.

Whether you are a young woman with a normal menstrual cycle or a more mature women who is menopausal, this program will take advantage of your hormonal state and teach you how to combine diet and exercise in just the right way.

What you have been taught in the male-dominated world of health and fitness is all wrong. It is time to get it right once and for all.

For a woman, it is not about working harder or longer or more often. That is the male approach, and it almost always results in overtraining. The female approach is to work smarter, not harder, to leverage your unique hormonal attributes in a way that harmonizes your health and fitness. This is what I am going to teach you.

I can't wait to see your changes. Let's get started.

HOW *METABOLIC RENEWAL* WORKS

Most people think exercising to burn fat is simply about working harder. It's not.

Most people think that optimizing your diet simply means eating less. That isn't true either

Eat less, exercise more. It's the conventional wisdom. The problem is, it doesn't work for most people in the long run. You can be as diligent and consistent as you like, but if you are working harder at the wrong things you are increasing your odds of failure, not success.

Most people view metabolism like it's a calculator—just punch in a lower number of calories consumed by eating less, and a higher number of calories burned by exercising more and voila, you'll lose weight. But it's more like one of those video games that reacts and gets more difficult the better you do.

You push on your metabolism by exercising harder or eating less, and what does your metabolism do? It pushes back, and makes you hungry and tired, increases cravings and saps your motivation. It adapts and reacts. You think you're burning more fat, but in reality you are setting yourself up for failure later on.

You know that old game you used to play when you were a kid, the one where you would try to run up an escalator that was going down? Imagine that escalator matching your speed and always staying one step ahead. You would be in for the ride of your life with nowhere to go but down. That is what following the standard diet and exercise advice will get you.

Exercise is not just about quantity. Longer is not better.

Diet is not just about quantity either. Less is not better.

And it's not a simple matter of quality either. Harder, shorter workouts don't guarantee success either. Better quality food is certainly important, but that alone won't shift the scales for good either. There is something else that is required. Something that determines whether or not your diet and exercise plan will make a difference in the way you look, feel and function.

Efficiency.

Fat-burning exercise is about efficiency. It is about doing the maximum amount of intelligent exercise in the shortest amount of time while adjusting to your specific fitness level. It's about eating in a realistic way—a way you can stick to for life—that accounts for your personal metabolic needs.

The most important word here is "intelligent." Intelligent exercise is exercise that provides just the right type of stimulus, in just the right amounts, to get your body to do what you want. Intelligent eating is sustainable and takes into account your individualized biochemistry and how it may react in unique ways to different foods.

How do you eat and exercise more intelligently as a woman? Well, you need to work with your unique female physiology. That means paying attention to your natural rhythms and how they impact your hormones, whether from changes in your menstrual cycle or as you progress through different stages of menopause. You need to understand your hormone type.

YOUR REPRODUCTIVE CYCLE DOES MAKE A DIFFERENCE

Does being a woman mean you should diet and exercise differently than men? In my opinion, yes. In fact, you should eat and exercise in a way that makes sense for your body and your hormone type. I'll get to what your hormone type is in a minute, but first let's look at why a female-specific approach is important.

Research into the metabolic effects of exercise has been dominated by the male perspective for years. This is mostly because, historically, exercise research has been geared toward young male athletes or fit college-aged males. This has changed in the last 30 to 40 years, but research into female metabolism still lags behind that of men.

It is commonly understood that men enjoy more muscle mass, greater strength and a lower percentage of body fat compared to women, largely due to testosterone. Men have higher resting levels of testosterone, and get a greater testosterone surge from exercise.

What you may not realize is that women also have hormonal advantages. Two of the most important are estrogen and HGH. Later in the program, I will explain in detail how balancing these and other hormones in your body can create the perfect environment for fat burning.

The key thing to understand now is that you, as a woman, have your own biochemical fat-burning advantage. But how do you access it? You need to understand your hormone type.

UNDERSTANDING YOUR HORMONE TYPE

Estrogen and progesterone influence nearly every other hormone in your body, including those involved in the speed of your metabolism, your ability to regulate blood sugar, and more. Of course, your estrogen and progesterone levels are, themselves, influenced by many things, including whether or not you are menstruating, which stage of menopause you're in, how you currently eat, exercise, live and more.

And here's another little secret that the weight loss community isn't telling you: A one-size-fits-all approach doesn't work—for anyone, really—but it is especially problematic for women, because they change hormonally and biochemically on a week-to-week and month-to-month basis throughout the course of their reproductive lives, and they change as they age, under stress or illness, and for many other reasons.

You need to take these factors into account if you want to burn fat and keep it off permanently. You need to stop thinking of metabolism as a calculator and get smart so you can react and adapt just as it does. You need to eat, exercise and live in a way that makes sense for where you are in your menstrual cycle and your time of life.

But if estrogen and progesterone levels fluctuate over the course of a woman's life, how do you know where you stand right now? How you can you design a program that is specific to your personal biochemistry if you don't even know what that is?

This is where your hormone type comes in. Understanding your hormone type is a convenient and efficient way to get a sense of where you are with estrogen and progesterone balance, which allows you to further customize this program to your unique female metabolism.

To help you identify your hormone type, I have developed a quiz that I will explain more about in a moment. First, I want you to understand one very important idea.

We humans can be funny creatures, and whenever someone says we are a particular "type" we get attached to that and start to believe it as gospel. This is the wrong way to view your hormone type. In reality, there is no great or definitive science that tells us what type you are. These types are just a clinical tool that I (and other doctors) use to help our patients get a general idea of how their metabolisms are operating at the current moment.

They are a starting point. They provide a very good structure for you to build on, but the major goal is for you to use them as a launching pad to discover your unique metabolic or hormone type. In reality, there is no such thing as a "hormone type" or a "metabolic type." There are infinite types and your job in this program is to discover yours.

The Hormone-Type Quiz will help you do that by giving you a nice starting point based on your current symptoms. The rest of the program will help you tweak, adjust, and manipulate four major metabolic parameters to fit your unique, specific needs.

HORMONE-TYPE QUIZ

To take the hormone-type quiz go to http://www.metabolicrenewal.com/quiz.

We built this quiz as an online tool only, because it is sophisticated and takes into account various factors about your life stage, cycle, environment and hormones to help develop an accurate picture of how your hormones and metabolism are currently operating.

Once you understand your hormone type, there are many things we can do to create a program specifically for your hormone type. When you think about making these adjustments to your metabolism, I want you to imagine a pyramid—a metabolic pyramid—and this pyramid has four main areas you can influence—the 4Ms.

WHAT ARE THE 4MS?

Metabolic Renewal draws on my 25 years of experience in health and fitness to deliver a program that does in 12 weeks what the programs I wrote a mere three years ago would have taken six months to accomplish.

I refer to the approach I've developed as the 4Ms. They are:

- ✓ Mindset or mindfulness (which helps combat stress)
- ✓ Movement (which controls stress and helps the body produce less fat-storing hormones)
- ✓ Meals (which help control calories and assures good nutrition)
- ✓ Metabolics (this is the stuff that stimulates and moves our metabolism like exercise, supplements and drugs)

Let me tell you a little about each part of the program.

Mindset

As I have already mentioned, women are typically more stress-reactive than men. That means the lifestyle portion of this program is absolutely critical.

One of the most frustrating things for any woman is to be doing everything right and feel like it's not working. Have you ever had that feeling when it comes to diet and exercise? Well, the clients I have worked with my entire career often feel this way when they first come to my clinic and they are often resistant to the truth of what is happening.

There are two reasons this happens. The first I have already explained: It has to do with the very wrong belief that you can follow an off-the-shelf, one-size-fits all program and magically see results. It does not work that way. You have to discover what works for you, and then design your own program built around that knowledge.

The second reason people can be doing everything right and not see results is a little bit harder to take. You see, body change is not just about diet and exercise. This is the reason you could be doing everything you think you are supposed to do and still see little for your effort.

Your metabolism is very much like a stress barometer and it measures more than just what you eat and how you exercise. Metabolism needs times to be fed, times to be without food, times to move intensely and most of all it needs time for rest and recovery. That last part is the most critical aspect of metabolic healing that everyone misses. They wrongly assume they can just work harder at diet and exercise and magically make a shift. I am here to tell you that this is wrong, wrong, wrong.

The most important part of this entire program is learning to live what I call a "rest-based lifestyle." One where you have plenty of recovery time.

We are talking about relaxing strolls through the park, a hot Epsom salt bath, supportive conversations with friends over coffee or wine, plenty of cuddling and sex (orgasm is incredibly healing to the metabolism), time with pets, (as long as they are not stressing you out,) naps, quality sleep, time at the spa and every other activity that lowers stress hormones and allows your metabolism to take a much needed relaxing sigh.

These behaviors are so important that I call them "rest and recovery workouts," because without them it does not matter what you eat or how much you exercise even if you are doing exactly what you have found works for you.

You must learn to chill the hell out.

When you do, you lower the constant onslaught of cortisol and other stress hormones in your body. Your hypothalamus and pituitary (the command and control center of your metabolism) start to rest and reboot your hormonal software. That's when the magic begins to happen.

You see, *Metabolic Renewal* is much more than a simple exercise or fat-loss program. It is meant to be a holistic, comprehensive guide to developing a way of eating, exercising and living that works for you. When you find that path, extraordinary things can happen.

In addition to burning fat, you may find that mood swings, cravings, cramps and bloating disappear. You may feel more energetic and focused than you have in a long time. You will be ready to tackle life again—maybe even in a way you never have before.

After all, life is short. We all want to make the most of it. This program will help you do that.

Movement

Science now tells us that exercise and movement should be thought of as slightly different things. In metabolic research, we have something I mentioned earlier that we call non-exercise associated thermogenesis (NEAT.) This constitutes all the movement you do in a day. Walking to the mailbox, taking the stairs, parking further away, doing the dishes, washing the laundry, gardening and everything else.

Believe it or not, this walking/movement impacts your metabolism 10% more than exercise does.[2] It's huge. And it helps balance estrogen and progesterone deficiency by helping the body reduce stress—walking lowers cortisol—and be less reactive to high-calorie foods, since it makes you more insulin-sensitive.

I'll go into more details about all of this in Chapter 10, which is dedicated to movement. For now, suffice it to say that daily movement is a tremendously important part of this program, and one of the healthiest things you can do.

Meals

In case you haven't noticed, you are not a man. Well, of course I know you know that, but the rest of the health and fitness world seems to forget it. However, you are also unique among women as well. You might be in your twenties, recently had your first child, going through the early stages of menopause or struggling with female specific metabolic issues like PCOS, hypothyroid or estrogen dominance.

This plan is built for you as a woman and as an individual.

You will learn how to adjust your eating, exercise and lifestyle to fit in with your monthly hormonal fluctuations if you are still menstruating. You will learn how to tackle the metabolic changes of pregnancy and menopause. You will learn how the modern-day stressors in your life can create metabolic challenges to which you may be especially susceptible.

One-size-fits-all programs do not work. You have to understand that, as a woman, you need to do things differently than a man. You also need to understand that not every woman can handle a diet and exercise program built for twenty-something female fitness competitors. You are a woman, yes, but you are a unique individual as well. In this program, you will learn how to stop trying to find "the right program" and instead build a diet, exercise routine and lifestyle that is perfectly suited to you and your hormone type.

I am going to teach you how to stop being a dieter and start being a metabolic detective. This way you will know how to deal with your current metabolism and also learn a tried and true process that will allow you to adjust to the metabolic changes every woman goes through, whether that's menstruation, stress, pregnancy, a damaged metabolism or menopause.

The end result will be a set of guidelines you will be able to tweak, mold, adjust and use to your advantage, working with, rather than against, your unique metabolic expression, psychology and personal preferences.

Metabolics

By "metabolics" I mean anything that stimulates or attempts to push on your metabolism. Remember, metabolism is an adaptive reactive system and that gives us the ability to try to "make it" do certain things.

We can exercise and try to stimulate the metabolism to burn fat or build muscle. We can take supplements to try to support a particular biochemical pathway. We can also take drugs to block or stimulate a certain biochemical reaction.

The metabolics category is important and powerful, but it works best under the right metabolic conditions. This is why it comes last in the 4Ms hierarchy. You can't out-train a poor diet. You can't expect to lose weight if you exercise but never move. And you can't sustain change in anything if you have not cultivated the right mindset and are mindful about stress. Metabolic stimulation is seductive for many because it "feels like" you are doing something, and you are. But it is only as powerful as the other 3Ms.

I have built the exercise portion of the program in four phases, each containing three workouts and each lasting three weeks. The workouts are just 15 minutes, three times a week, and the exercises are just 45 seconds each. They're hyper-efficient and hyper-effective, helping you to burn fat, tone muscle and stay young. That's it. Simple, but powerful.

Each phase is designed to gradually upgrade your body and your metabolism, enhancing your nerves, muscles, coordination, strength and conditioning in a safe and methodical way. So many women try to do too much too soon without properly preparing their bodies, at which point your metabolism fights back, forcing weight gain and energy loss. That won't happen with *Metabolic Renewal*'s strategically-designed, gradual, phased approach.

Here is what you can expect in each phase.

PHASE 1: HARMONIZE

This phase is all about getting your hormonal system back into balance and harmony. We do this by working on the command and control centers of your metabolism, the hypothalamus and pituitary gland, areas of the brain that govern your metabolism, reaction to stress and more.

Why is this important?

Women are typically more stress-reactive than men. From an evolutionary standpoint this makes sense, as they are the reproductive gender. The body needs to be very clear if it's under too much stress to safely have a baby or not. So the hypothalamus and pituitary gland in women is hypersensitive.

The problem is that in the modern world, most women are overstressed. Over-exercising, extreme dieting, sleep deprivation, not to mention the daily stresses of a career, parenting and more, cause a lot of women to be very stressed out. This sends your whole metabolism out of control, because it impacts you at a deep biochemical level. Since your hypothalamus and pituitary are responsible for hormonal balance, you can imagine what happens when they aren't functioning properly. Hormonal messages either don't get released or don't get communicated effectively, and your entire metabolism breaks down at the very root.

We need to manage that stress and rebalance the body if we are going to help you burn fat. We need to rebalance your hormones, and make sure your little cellular messengers are delivering their messages properly. We need to get you ready for the more intense exercise that is to come. Which is precisely what Phase 1 does.

In the beginning, you may feel a little off balance or be unsure about the movements. This is normal and by design. In fact, in this phase I purposely expose you to exercise and movement patterns that challenge you differently than other types of exercise, specifically so we can stress the body in a systematic way to prepare it for the next phase.

You will soon learn that there are four critical components of the *Metabolic Renewal* workout. I call them the Bs and Hs. They are:

- ✓ **Breathless**
- ✓ **Burning**
- ✓ **Heavy**
- ✓ **Heat**

I'll explain more about why these Bs and Hs are so important for a high-intensity workout in Chapter 8. For now, just be aware that this program hits all four of them, but it specifically focuses on "breathless" and "burning" because these are the two biochemical feedback signals that indicate that you are taking advantage of your unique female fat-loss advantage.

You can think of this like an athlete going into spring training. You will be getting the metabolic benefits from day one, but we also have to lay the metabolic framework and rebalance your hormones so you can benefit maximally from Phases 2, 3 and 4.

PHASE 2: INSPIRE

Once your hormones and the control and command center of your brain are rebalanced, the next step is to get your cells ready to receive the messages being sent.

This helps turn on your metabolism's ability to burn fat for energy, giving you the metabolic flexibility to burn either carbs or fat for energy based on what your body needs at the time. That's important because most women (and men) are stuck with metabolisms that can mostly only burn carbs for energy, causing them to eat frequently and suffer from major ups and down of energy. Adding the ability to burn fat allows you to eat less while stabilizing your energy.

Think of your hormones like mail carriers—they carry messages around the body. But the cells need to receive these messages if your metabolism is to function correctly. Phase 2 inspires your cells to wake up, clearing out the cobwebs that are gumming up your cellular machinery right now. It increases receptor sensitivity at the cellular level, meaning your metabolic mail carrier (your hormones) can deliver their messages more efficiently and effectively.

This impacts your metabolism all the way down to the mitochondrial level. Your mitochondria are the little powerhouses in your cells that burn fat and create energy. If your cells can't get messages from your hormones, your mitochondria won't function optimally.

That means reduced fat loss, reduced energy, poor mood and more. So in this phase we ramp things up a little bit to prevent that problem. We get your cells inspired to "hear" the fat burning messages they receive.

PHASE 3: ENHANCE

Now that we have your hormones rebalanced and your cells ready to hear their messages, it's time to turn up the heat. At this point in the program your body will be better able to handle the stress hormones that are so important to enhancing the effects of exercise.

Did I just say stress hormones can be a good thing?

I did, and they can. You see, your stress hormones—the catecholamines—are a critical component of the fat-burning hormonal cocktail. They aren't inherently bad. In fact, under the right circumstances, they can have a tremendous positive impact on your fat-burning metabolism.

The problem is that most of us are too stressed out too much of the time, our hormones are out of balance, and our cellular machinery isn't functioning properly. When you add more stress in a situation like this—even otherwise healthy stress like exercise—you can set the stage for disaster.

But in the last two phases we have systematically upgraded your metabolism to handle more and more intense exercise, which is exactly what you are going to get in Phase 3. This phase will leave you breathless—a very good sign that it is doing its job, releasing those catecholamines, and burning up fat like crazy.

PHASE 4: SYMPHONY

This is where the rubber meets the road. Your hormones have been harmonized, your cells inspired, and you've enhanced your fat-burning machinery. Now it's time to bring the entire metabolic symphony together so it can play its beautiful music.

Phase 4 is a culmination of all the work we've done in the last three phases. The big metabolic benefit is that you will be taking advantage of your unique female ability to tap into and use human growth hormone (HGH).

You see, women release more HGH in response to exercise than men do, and this is a very good thing. HGH is the primary metabolic multitasker, enhancing the effects of all the other fat-burning, muscle-sculpting hormones in the body. It delivers its muscle-shaping messages by amplifying the effects of estrogen and testosterone in building and tightening lean muscle.

But unlike testosterone, HGH won't make you bulky. It's responsible for lean muscle, not bulky muscle, so you won't start looking like Arnold Schwarzenegger. HGH also happens to impact collagen, which means your skin may look healthier and tighter than it has in decades—one of the wonderful side benefits you will get from the *Metabolic Renewal* program.

By the time Phase 4 is over, your metabolism will be functioning on a whole other level. It will be completely different from where it was when you started. It will be renewed. That means that you will not only burn fat and shape lean muscles, you will reinvigorate your body and feel healthier than you have in a long time.

Speaking of health, let's take a few minutes to look at some of the health benefits, aside from fat burning, that you are bound to experience on this program.

METABOLIC RENEWAL AND YOUR HEALTH

It is important to remember that looking good and feeling better are not the only things *Metabolic Renewal* will help you accomplish. It will also help you get healthier and live longer. If there is one thing exercise excels at, it is extending the quality and quantity of life.

The strategies we use for the nutrition, exercise and lifestyle components of *Metabolic Renewal* have repeatedly been shown in multiple studies to enhance health, protect you from chronic disease, and even reverse the progress of some illnesses. What follows is not a comprehensive review of the health benefits of the program. It's just a sample to show you what a powerful effect *Metabolic Renewal* has, not only your fitness levels, but also on your overall health.

Ultimately, you want to look good, feel good and live longer. I want to take a brief moment to point out to you some of the amazing science we now have on how short, intense workouts like the ones you will do in this program can not only reduce the risk of disease, but also treat it.

The biggest health concerns for most of the women I have worked with are heart disease, cancer, diabetes and brain and memory concerns like Alzheimer's.

Cardiovascular Disease

Cardiovascular disease is the leading killer of both women and men, and I want you to know that the workout you will be doing in *Metabolic Renewal* is incredibly powerful at helping to keep your heart healthy.

One of my favorite studies to demonstrate this was published in 2007 in the highly respected journal *Circulation*.[3] This study compared interval-style training to standard aerobic training in about 20 patients with heart failure.

I realize that you may not have heart failure, but that is why I like this study so much. If this style of exercise can help those with the most unhealthy hearts, it can definitely help you. The patients received three workouts a week for 12 weeks and then were compared one to the other.

While both groups saw improvements, the interval group saw more benefits in almost all the areas examined. What was most striking was the interval workout's ability to impact left ventricular remodeling. This is a measure of how efficient and functional the heart is. The workout using intense bursts followed by rest actually improved heart function, while the traditional workout had no effect.

This same study showed improvements in cholesterol, blood pressure and blood-flow kinetics as well.

Cancer

Cancer is typically cited as the second-leading cause of death among women. Like cardiovascular disease, some believe cancer to be a disease of poor lifestyle. It is widely recognized that exercise in general reduces the risk of cancer, but do high-intensity workouts using rest intervals have any special effects in this realm?

It appears these types of workouts may have an advantage here as well. Again, I like to quote studies of those already dealing with the issue. My rationale is that if the workout helps those already diagnosed, it should be even more beneficial for those not yet dealing with cancer.

In a study, 24 women were prescribed a similar type of workout to *Metabolic Renewal* two years after cancer diagnosis. They were followed for 12 weeks, did three workouts a week, and were randomized to either a short-burst and then rest group or a traditional aerobic group.

The interval group exercised for 20 minutes, although only 3.5 minutes of that time was work, the remainder was active rest (similar to the slow walking you do during the Renewal workouts). The traditional cardio group worked out for 30 minutes and all 30 minutes were work.

The interval group outperformed the traditional aerobic group in most all parameters studied, including increased fitness, quality of life scores, and most importantly, enjoyability of the workout.

This study was published in the October 2016 issue of the journal *PeerJ*.[4]

Type 2 Diabetes

Type 2 diabetes is an interesting condition because most doctors agree that it is an issue itself, but also increases the risk of the two major killers of women: heart disease and cancer.

In a study, 28 diabetes patients were followed for 12 weeks to assess the outcomes of a short duration, high-intensity workout utilizing rest. The study was published in 2016 in Volume 59 of one of the most prestigious journals specializing in diabetes: *Diabetologia*.[5]

This study involved a mix of cardio bursts and weight lifting exercises very similar to what you are doing in the *Metabolic Renewal* workouts. The participants exercised only three times per week.

The workout produced some pretty substantial changes. Blood sugar levels improved, abdominal fat decreased and liver function—a major issue in diabetics—improved substantially.

Brain Health

When I talk to my female patients who are around the age of forty, they invariably admit their fear about decreasing brain function as they age. Alzheimer's is one of those conditions that makes all of my patients a little worried.

So will *Metabolic Renewal* help your brain? According to a 2014 article in the *Journal of Rehabilitation Medicine*, it definitely does.[6]

Obese subjects were put on a workout regime that combined short bursts of activity followed by rest with circuit weight training. *Metabolic Renewal* uses a similar approach, combining both of these modalities into a single workout.

After four months brain function—as measured by short-term and working memory, attention and processing speed, and long-term verbal memory—was significantly improved. Some of these parameters improved by over 30%.

Musculoskeletal Health

If you asked me what I thought the number one killer of women and men is, I would say frailty. The reason? Those who have strong physical bodies fare much better when they get sick and are more likely to recover. A strong woman who falls will be less likely to break a hip. If she does, she will be more likely to recover.

You may be aware of this, but hip fractures are fairly common in women as they age, and can be a deadly event due to severe complications.

Exercise of all types helps the bone, muscle and nervous system, which are all required to keep you from falling and minimize damage if you do. But do *Metabolic Renewal* workouts do a better job than traditional workouts?

Yes, they do. Not only do weight-training workouts like this help burn fat and build bone, they help you become stronger and more flexible. The combination of strong and flexible is the holy grail of muscle and bone health.

A 12-week weight training program not only increased bone mineral density by 2.1%, something that research has shown no other type of exercise can do, it also increased flexibility by 150% compared to traditional stretching. I bet that puts an entirely new spin on what type of exercise you should be doing for flexibility, doesn't it?

These two studies were published in the April 2014 and December 2011 issues of *The Strength and Conditioning Journal* (my favorite journal).[7,8]

There are, of course, a ton of other benefits to this type of training. There are thousands of studies demonstrating the impact of this type of workout on health parameters. I provided some of my favorite studies and addressed some of the major concerns I know women wonder about.

You may not be a science nerd like me, but I hope this gives you the confidence to know that you are doing something great for your body. You also may want to share this information with your doctor, so he or she knows that you are in good hands and using a scientifically sound, evidence-based workout program.

Alright, now that we've laid the foundation, let's start digging into the juicy details and talk about why *Metabolic Renewal* works the way it does. I can't think of a better place to start than the three laws of metabolism.

WHAT YOU LEARNED IN THIS CHAPTER:

✓ "Eat less, exercise more" doesn't work for most people.

✓ You need to diet and exercise smarter, not harder.

✓ Your cycle and your hormone type have a tremendous influence on your ability to burn fat, and this program will teach you how to leverage that advantage.

✓ There are 4Ms when it comes to fat loss: mindset, movement, meals, and metabolics. Historically, diet programs have focused too much on diet and exercise to the exclusion of the others.

✓ Better diet and exercise is ultimately about pulling specific metabolic and hormonal triggers that will reprogram your body to burn fat.

✓ *Metabolic Renewal* achieves this by utilizing a technique called rest-based training that allows you to tailor each exercise session to your personal physiology and needs, and it provides a customizable dietary program you can fit to your own needs as woman.

✓ It is a 12-week, four-phase program that will systematically provide you with a metabolic makeover.

✓ The plan also has a wide variety of positive effects on your health.

✓ Despite what you might have heard, when it comes to exercise, men and women are different. This program is designed specifically to give women a hormonal advantage.

THE THREE LAWS OF METABOLISM

When it comes to fitness, harder is not better, smarter is better.

Metabolic Renewal is a better program because it changes the key metabolic hormones that act as the control switch for fat burning. Other programs focus on calories first. This program focuses on metabolic balance first. I am going to teach you exactly how it works.

But before you can understand why this program works so well, we have to cover some basic rules of fat loss. We will call these the three laws of metabolism.

#1: THE LAW OF METABOLIC COMPENSATION

Some people compare the metabolism to a calculator. Others compare it to a chemistry lab. Both of these models are wrong. There is no standard math equation or chemical recipe that unlocks fat loss.

The metabolism is most like a thermostat or seesaw. It adjusts and responds in the opposite direction to stimuli, always seeking balance. This is why when you eat less and exercise more, your metabolism will produce changes that make it so you will compensate with more hunger, lower energy, increased cravings and a slower metabolic rate. All these changes ensure that you will soon end up eating more, exercising less and regain any lost fat and possibly more.

When your sleep, hunger, mood, energy and cravings—what I call SHMEC (pronounced "shmeck")—are out of balance, you know that the law of metabolic compensation is working against you. Smarter, more intelligent programs work with, rather than against, this metabolic compensation. They keep your SHMEC in check and your metabolism humming. You will learn why in a minute.

#2: THE LAW OF METABOLIC MULTITASKING

The two dominant models for body change are "eat like a bird and run for miles" and "eat less carbs and more protein plus lift weights."

The first approach burns fat, but also breaks down muscle. The result is you get smaller but flabbier. What is often referred to as "skinny fat." The second approach builds or maintains muscle, but does little to burn fat. This results in a bigger, more bulky appearance. When you gain muscle under a layer of fat that is not burned, it is like putting a jacket on top of two sweaters. Of course, you look bulky.

The body likes to be burning or building, and does not do well managing both at the same time. That's why you see athletes or more advanced fitness buffs do separate workouts for cardio to burn fat and weight training to build muscle. There's just one problem—that burns up a lot of time we probably don't have given that we're all juggling competing priorities at work and at home and struggling to find the time to really do anything consistently for ourselves.

Smarter programs primarily burn fat, and utilize special metabolic tactics that shape and firm muscle as well. You are going to learn exactly how this program accomplishes both. It'll save you a ton of time and deliver results that you can both see and feel surprisingly quickly.

#3: THE LAW OF METABOLIC EFFICIENCY AND INDIVIDUALITY

Your metabolism is not wasteful, and, as you have learned, is highly reactive to changes. Doing more exercise or longer exercise can easily become a stress to the body, especially if you are just starting out. Eating less while exercising more only worsens the problem.

When your body is stressed you create the opposite changes from what you are after. Rather than getting a faster, healthier metabolism with less fat and better muscle tone, you will get a slower, more sluggish metabolism with more fat and flabby muscles.

Efficiency is the name of the game when it comes to finding the sweet spot of health and fitness. I call this the Goldilocks effect. You don't want too much or too little. You want it just right.

This program combines optimal intensity that is individualized to you, with short, directed exercise sessions. Its nutrition plan is built so that it can be tailored to your needs, and the focus on rest-based living gives you the structure and space to cool down stress overall. You do just the right amount to get the result, but not too much to throw your metabolism out of balance.

The three laws of metabolism have to be honored if you want to make sure you burn fat and keep it off. Violating these laws for any length of time almost ensures rebound fat gain and wasted effort. *Metabolic Renewal* works with these three laws to make sure your metabolism stays balanced, SHMEC stays in check and you slowly build your body into a fat-burning furnace.

One of the chief ways it does this is by paying special attention to your hormonal balance. After all, your hormones have a tremendous impact on your metabolism. Most women know this. They realize hormones impact fat-burning. But here's the secret: The most important hormones for fat-burning are not the ones you think they are.

WHAT YOU LEARNED IN THIS CHAPTER:

✓ There are three laws of metabolism that constitute the basic rules for how you burn fat.

✓ Law #1 tells us that your metabolism is more like a thermostat or seesaw than a calculator. It adjusts and responds to your diet and lifestyle. This is why the classic "eat less, exercise more" advice for weight loss doesn't work.

✓ Law #2 tells us that your metabolism doesn't like to multitask. It likes to be building or burning, not both. This is why we must trick your body with specialized metabolic techniques that will allow you build or shape muscle while burning fat at the same time.

✓ Law #3 tells us that your metabolism is not wasteful. Efficiency is the name of the game. This is why you want neither too much nor too little exercise.

✓ These three laws must be obeyed if you want to burn fat and keep it off.

3

IS IT REALLY ALL ABOUT HORMONES?

Most women know instinctually that their hormones influence their weight. But here's the thing, it's not the hormones you think.

Yes, it is true that estrogen and progesterone—the hormones most intimately related to your menstrual cycle—are important. But what many women think is that estrogen and progesterone are the most important fat-burning and fat-storing hormones. They aren't. Insulin, cortisol, thyroid and your adrenals are all more important when it comes to fat loss.

In fact, estrogen and progesterone constitute the smallest part of what I call the Female Hormonal Triad. Here's an easy way to understand it:

At the base of the pyramid are insulin and cortisol. These are the primary hormones that influence your ability to burn fat. Just above them are thyroid and your adrenals. Then, all the way at the top—at the very smallest part of the pyramid—are estrogen and progesterone.

Why are they all the way at the top? Because they are not as important as the others, but they do influence each of the other hormones.

You see, your hormones all play together like a symphony. When one part of the symphony overwhelms another part, it impacts the

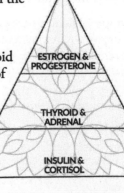

ESTROGEN &
PROGESTERONE

THYROID &
ADRENAL

INSULIN &
CORTISOL

harmony of the whole thing. And, like in a symphony, the instruments (in this case hormones) can have different effects. Sometimes they work one way, sometimes another, just like a violin can make you feel happy one moment and melancholy the next.

The best symphonies play in tune together. They are balanced, and that is exactly what you want with your hormones. Again, this is all about the Goldilocks effect. Not too little and not too much—but just right.

Of course, calories matter too. If they were pictured here, they would share the base of the pyramid with insulin and cortisol. However, if you get your hormones right, often the calories take care of themselves.

I don't want to write a textbook on hormones here. But I do want you to understand how some of the key hormones—including your female hormones—impact your ability to burn fat.

INSULIN: THE FAT STORER

In the hierarchy of hormonal influencers for fat loss, insulin still reigns as king. This hormone, relative to the others, is most strongly influenced by carbohydrate intake and overconsumption of food, both of which cause a detrimental increase in blood sugar.

For the average American who tends to be sedentary and also over consumes, insulin will increase and remain high. Chronic high levels of insulin will eventually cause your body to become resistant to this hormone, meaning you will have difficulty burning fat.

With the epidemic of Type 2 diabetes and obesity, this means that most Americans are insulin resistant and thus unable to burn fat. Interestingly, estrogen makes you more insulin-sensitive. As you age, estrogen naturally declines until you reach menopause, when it plummets and your whole female physiology changes. Think about what that means when it comes to your cycle and time of life.

As these hormones fluctuate over the course of your menstrual cycle and as you move through various phases of life—from normal menstruation to compromised menstruation for some to pregnancy and eventually menopause—you will become more or less insulin sensitive as your levels of estrogen and progesterone rise and fall. This program takes into account this fluctuation allowing you to maximize your results by taking advantage of these changes instead of falling victim to them.

CORTISOL: THE STRESS HORMONE

Cortisol, secreted from the adrenal glands, has a split personality in the body. In other words, it is not all bad or all good. Acute stressors on the body tend to cause a short-term increase of this hormone. It gets the body primed to either fight or flee from the stress. This served us well in the Paleolithic era when we were not at the top of the food chain.

A lion jumping out at us requires metabolic messengers that are quick acting to prime us to fight or flee for our lives. Cortisol, along with adrenaline, serves this purpose. Once we get out of danger, these hormones allow us to get stronger and better for the next time a predator thinks we are food. Unfortunately, these days our hectic lifestyles cause our adrenal glands to think there are dangerous creatures everywhere jumping out at us, thus cortisol levels tend to be either chronically elevated or very, very low, both of which can create a fatty, fatigued body.

Interestingly, estrogen and progesterone both cause cortisol to be less detrimental. When levels fall you become more sensitive to cortisol and its negative effects, which is one of the reasons women are more stress reactive. However, that also means that there are certain times in your life and in your cycle when you are super buffered against cortisol. As you'll see in this program, you can take advantage of this fact to get even better results.

THYROID: THE METABOLIC MANAGER

Thyroid hormone, secreted from the thyroid gland, helps to manage the body's metabolic processes, including your fat-burning potential. It is like the thermostat on your metabolism. This hormone is also keenly sensitive to your daily lifestyle choices, including sleep (how long and how deep), nutrition (types and amounts), stress (acute or chronic) and exercise (longer moderate-intensity or shorter higher-intensity.)

Unfortunately, your thyroid gland is primed to think food will be scarce like it tended to be long ago in prehistoric times. This is why when someone goes on an "eat less and exercise more" program your thyroid will cause your body to slow down its metabolism.

If you've experience rebound weight gain after dieting, this may very well be why. When you eat less, your thyroid slows down to accommodate the reduction in calories. Then, when you go back to a regular diet, your metabolism is still operating in this downregulated state. Think about that: You're eating the same calories you did before your diet, but now your metabolism is burning even fewer calories than it did before. That's the perfect storm for fat gain, making fat loss next to impossible.

Estrogen and thyroid hormone have a special relationship. Higher than normal levels of estrogen increase a thyroid-binding hormone called TBG. High levels of TBG make thyroid less effective. So while estrogen levels that are too low are not a good thing, estrogen levels that are too high can negatively impact thyroid hormone production as well.

I know all of this can get a little confusing, but it will all make sense soon. For now just realize that when thinking about hormones you don't want too much or too little, but levels that are just right, like Goldilocks.

THE ADRENALS: THE METABOLIC GAS PEDAL

Epinephrine and norepinephrine, referred to as catecholamines, along with cortisol, get secreted by the adrenal glands any time you are stressed. This happens especially when you exercise. The great thing about the catecholamines is that they tell the body to get ready to start burning fat.

But again, too much of a good thing is not healthy for the female metabolism, which likes balance. When it comes to the catecholamines, you want them elevated during exercise, but turned off during rest. This is going to be a recurring theme throughout this program and why the section on rest-based living is going to be so important for you to master.

These catecholamines also signal to other hormones, like HGH, cortisol and testosterone, encouraging them to go into fat burning mode. As you might imagine, the catecholamines have a close working relationship with cortisol, given they are both secreted from the adrenal gland. Their effects can be blunted if cortisol levels are not optimal.

And, as we saw with insulin and thyroid, estrogen and progesterone have an influence on adrenal hormones as well. They do this by blunting the negative effects of cortisol and other stress hormones.

ESTROGEN: FAT-LOSS HORMONE OR FAT-GAIN HORMONE?

Estrogen is a growth hormone. It's primarily responsible for the growth of the breasts and the uterine lining, but it plays a role in growth throughout the female body and can even impact the growth of muscle, brain cells, and other areas. So, estrogen is not just about reproduction; it's also about healthy growth all over the female metabolism.

Estrogen is an interesting hormone from the standpoint of weight loss and fat loss, because it causes weight loss globally but may cause fat gain locally on specific parts of the body. There is some evidence[9] showing that estrogen amplifies the number and activity of alpha-adrenergic receptors. These special fat cell regulators are concentrated in the lower body of women, especially in the hips, butt and thighs.

These receptors are responsible for slowing the release of fat, so stimulating their activity can slow down fat loss. This is one of the reasons estrogen causes women to have that beautiful hourglass shape. It keeps their waist smaller and their hips, bust, butt and thighs fuller.

At the same time, these receptors are also the reason many women lose weight faster from certain parts of the body than others. If estrogen levels and other hormones are not attended to, women can develop other, less flattering, shapes, like the pear or apple shape.

Similarly, these receptors explain why shape change can be so difficult, and why many women go from a large pear or apple shape to a smaller but more pronounced pear or apple shape, when they follow traditional diets. They restrict calories, but do nothing to impact hormones, and lack of real shape change is the reward.

This is also why measuring your hourglass shape (which you will do in this program) is a critical indicator of your estrogen and progesterone levels and balance. You can learn more about that in the bonus *The Metabolic Renewal Transformation Tracker.*

Estrogen may have the opposite effect on visceral adipose tissue or VAT. This is the fat that lies deep inside your body. It's not that stuff you can pinch an inch of. It's fat that surrounds your organs, especially your liver. Estrogen helps you effectively burn this fat, because it controls the two major hormones that store it—insulin and cortisol. That is why optimizing estrogen levels—not too much or too little—keeps you healthy and sexy.

It's also worth mentioning again that estrogen can negatively impact the action of thyroid. That means if you have too much estrogen your whole metabolism could slow down, leading to many negative downstream consequences beyond weight gain, including hypothyroidism.

In fact, estrogen dominance is an increasingly common problem—one that I talk about more below. But too little estrogen isn't good either, and here's why. Estrogen makes the

THE PROBLEM WITH HORMONE REPLACEMENT THERAPY

This idea of hormonal balance is one of the most important lessons you can take from this program. Hormones influence each other and your metabolism in complex ways.

It's almost never just about one hormone or another, but how the whole symphony plays together.

This is especially important for women, because during menopause or when you are metabolically challenged, the conventional wisdom says, "re-establish estrogen and progesterone and you'll start losing weight."

The traditional way to do that? Hormone replacement therapy or HRT.

I've seen hundreds of women come through my clinic on HRT, and in my experience it rarely works the way they want it to.

Why?

Synthetic hormones dock on your cellular receptors differently than natural ones do. And these hormones aren't delivered cyclically the way they naturally occur in your body.

When you don't take into account the hormonal hierarchy and the hormonal symphony, and simply use HRT to solve your problems, it usually doesn't work.

female metabolism more insulin-sensitive and less stress-reactive. You'll recall that insulin and cortisol are at the very base of our hormonal hierarchy for fat loss. If you are more insulin-sensitive and less stress-reactive, this is a very good thing for your body composition.

This is one of the key reasons young women who menstruate normally have an easier time burning fat and keeping it off than women in menopause or those who are metabolically challenged do.

When estrogen drops at the time of menopause, fat distribution changes, and women are more likely to gain weight, especially right around the middle. If you are metabolically challenged and dealing with a condition like PCOS, your hormones may fluctuate all over the place, making it very difficult to maintain the balance needed to burn fat and keep it off.

But there are ways you can better manage these situations. I'll show you how in this program.

PROGESTERONE: ESTROGEN'S UNRECOGNIZED STEPSISTER

Progesterone doesn't get the attention it deserves. But estrogen and progesterone are like sisters. They need each other. They balance each other out. Unfortunately, many people think of progesterone as the unrecognized or even the "ugly" stepsister in this equation. To me, this is the wrong way to think about progesterone.

If estrogen sends the "growth signals" to the breast, uterine lining and other areas, progesterone comes along and says, "Okay, not too much growth." Remember, it's all about Goldilocks here.

But progesterone has other effects as well, particularly on stress. When progesterone is out of balance, the first thing we see is women becoming more reactive to stress. Stress can cause drops in progesterone, which can cause a maladaptive stress response, creating a vicious cycle. When a woman is stressed out, this is usually how it is reflected in the metabolism.

Remember that stress leads to more cortisol, and chronically high-cortisol levels have a serious impact on fat gain. Progesterone can help blunt that effect if it is balanced. Unlike estrogen, progesterone has little to no direct effect on insulin. But it does influence it indirectly, because it opposes the action of estrogen. As you know, estrogen makes you more insulin sensitive. Since progesterone opposes the action of estrogen, it can make you more insulin resistant if it is too high for too long.

This is obviously not a good thing, because insulin resistance can lead to weight gain.

The important takeaway when it comes to progesterone is that it impacts fat loss or fat gain indirectly, due to how it influences cortisol and, more importantly, its balancing effects on estrogen. Estrogen and progesterone are important. But they are not your most important fat-burning hormones. That said, they do influence your most important fat-burning hormones, and that means you can mitigate any negative effects they have on your fat-burning potential by learning to live, eat and exercise in a way that is in tune with your hormone type.

To do that you need to understand a little more about your specific hormone type and how it influences your metabolism.

WHAT YOU LEARNED IN THIS CHAPTER:

✓ Estrogen and progesterone do impact fat loss, but not in the way you may have thought.

✓ They are not your primary fat-loss hormones, but they are important.

✓ Insulin, cortisol, thyroid and adrenals are also essential.

✓ Insulin is the king of fat loss hormones. Estrogen makes you more insulin sensitive.

✓ Cortisol can also lead to fat gain. Estrogen and progesterone protect you against it.

✓ Thyroid is like the gas pedal on your metabolism. It defines the speed at which it runs. Balanced female hormones affect thyroid positively.

✓ Adrenals also play a role in stress and fat gain. Estrogen and progesterone protect you against them.

✓ Estrogen is related to fat loss in complex ways. It may actually cause fat retention in certain tissues like the butt, hips, thighs and breast. But it helps you burn belly fat.

✓ Progesterone is estrogen's sister. It doesn't impact fat loss directly, but indirectly through its effect on cortisol and estrogen.

UNDERSTANDING YOUR HORMONE TYPE

All women experience the hormonal fluctuations that go along with menses and the changes that occur during a regular menstrual cycle, through pregnancy, and then through menopause. Even if you don't menstruate regularly or are somehow hormonally or metabolically challenged, you most likely remember a time your cycle was stable and smooth.

But not all women are aware of the precise way that estrogen, progesterone and other hormones ebb and flow. This is important because these hormones influence all of the other hormones in your body, especially your fat-burning hormones.

Your hormone type has a tremendous influence on your overall metabolic balance. These hormones, in turn, impact your metabolism. However, you can influence them based on how you eat, exercise, manage stress and move. This turns what is normally seen as a fat-burning disadvantage for women into a kind of female "superpower." But to take advantage of it, you need to know a little bit more about your specific hormone type.

IMPORTANT: I encourage you to read this whole chapter even if a specific hormone type doesn't apply to you. Your hormonal balance and hormone type are bound to change over time, maybe even over the course of this program. Understanding the different types will arm you with critical information you need as these changes occur.

All of you should read the section on the normal menstrual cycle, unless you are already very well versed in the biology of menses. Understanding the basic mechanics of female menstruation will inform everything you read in the rest of this program.

NORMAL MENSTRUAL CYCLE— ESTROGEN AND PROGESTERONE BALANCED

The menstrual cycle begins with the first day of menses or bleeding. About halfway through (day 14) ovulation occurs. The egg is then available for insemination for an additional 14 days, and the cycle repeats. For the first 14 days of your menstrual cycle, progesterone is relatively flat. In fact, young women have similar amounts of progesterone in their body as men do prior to ovulation. During this time estrogen slowly rises and peaks right around ovulation.

At this point in your cycle, you have more estrogen in your body relative to progesterone. This is called the "follicular" phase of your cycle, because this is when the follicle that hosts the egg begins to develop. Two other important hormones influence the development of the follicle: follicle-stimulating hormone (FSH) and luteinizing hormone (LH).

Toward the end of the follicular phase of the cycle (right around day 14), you experience a spike in LH. This causes the follicle to rupture and the egg to be released. During this same period, the uterine lining begins to thicken under the influence of estrogen.

Once ovulation occurs, and the egg is released, what's left of the follicle becomes the corpus luteum, which is the source of the name of the next part of the cycle: the "luteal phase." The corpus luteum becomes the source of progesterone. So, progesterone starts to rise and estrogen starts to fall after ovulation. Midway through the luteal phase you end up with more progesterone than estrogen. There is still a lot of estrogen around, but it's not dominant as it was before.

If the egg is not fertilized and implanted (attached to the wall of the uterus), progesterone and estrogen levels fall and the uterine lining is shed. Bleeding commences, and the cycle starts over.

WHAT IS PMS?

Premenstrual syndrome is believed to occur due to falling levels of either estrogen and/or progesterone in the week leading up to menses.

It is important to remember that there are receptors for estrogen and progesterone all over the body, including the brain, breast, muscle and fat cells.

One theory about what causes PMS in some women are levels of estrogen that are *always* a bit more prevalent than progesterone.

Female metabolism is exquisitely balanced in its cyclical fluctuations of estrogen and progesterone. Any change in this system—usually due to poorly designed diets or poor stress management—can result in symptoms of poor metabolic function.

As a result, SHMEC can go out of check and other uncomfortable symptoms can manifest including anxiety, depression, breast tenderness, cramping and other symptoms.

If you are a woman who has dealt with PMS, realize that this is a clue that your hormonal system may be out of balance, and you will want to use these symptoms as clues, like a detective, about how to design your new lifestyle in this program.

As you make progress, you may be surprised to see that these symptoms begin to dramatically improve.

I know that may seem a bit complicated, so here's a graphic that illustrates this process.

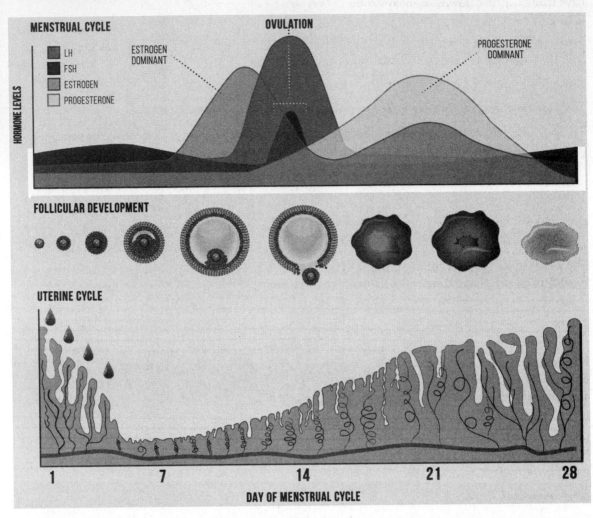

As you can see, there is a natural ebb and flow of estrogen and progesterone throughout the cycle. This is important to understand, so I'm going to say it again: The first 14 days of your cycle is a time of more estrogen relative to progesterone. Then, after ovulation, there is a time of more progesterone than estrogen. Both hormones are still high, but progesterone dominates.

This ebb and flow of hormones, and the way it fluctuates throughout the life of a woman (from pregnancy through menopause), causes all the changes associated with female metabolism.

What this means is that if you learn to live, eat and exercise in harmony with your hormones, you can take your fat-burning potential to a whole new level.

NORMAL MENSTRUAL CYCLE—ESTROGEN DOMINANT

Estrogen dominance occurs when you have too much estrogen relative to progesterone for too long. A younger woman who menstruates normally will be estrogen dominant in the first half of her cycle and progesterone dominant in the second half of her cycle. This is not a problem. In fact, this ebb and flow of hormones is exactly as nature intended. However, if you remain estrogen dominant for too long it can have many negative downstream consequences on your health, including fat gain.

You should know there are really no good measurements for this that you can get at your doctor's office. Estrogen dominance is what we call a "clinical manifestation"—it makes sense, it is consistent with the science, but we don't have an accurate way of measuring it.

Estrogen dominance can occur for many reasons. Let's take a look at a few of them.

You Remain Estrogen Dominant Throughout Your Cycle

This can happen for many reasons, including not ovulating. Since the corpus luteum is the source of progesterone, and it is only formed if ovulation occurs, lack of ovulation means no progesterone. The two major reasons this happens are stress and menopause. In fact, a young woman undergoing a lot of stress can push her metabolism into a state that closely resembles menopause.

It is useful to remind yourself that your female metabolism is exquisitely tuned to stress reactions. This is a requirement since your metabolism is built to prepare you for an optimal pregnancy. If it were not for the female metabolism's ability to finely tune itself to stressors, the human race would not have fared very well.

Too much stress, whether through chronic dieting, extreme exercise or any other source, will register in your metabolism and disrupt the natural rhythm of estrogen and progesterone, leading to lack of ovulation and all the downstream negative effects.

Stress

Chronic stress can place younger women in a menopause-like state too. This happens for many complex biochemical reasons, but here is the short version. Chronic stress "agitates" the hypothalamus-pituitary-ovarian axis. This is the highway of information that runs from your brain to your reproductive organs and governs the whole process of menstruation and ovulation.

When there is too much traffic on this highway, or the traffic is "driving like crazy," it causes changes in FSH and LH, and therefore can impact ovulation in ways that are similar to what we see in menopause. If a young woman is presenting with menopause-like symptoms, it's almost always a sign that she is under extreme stress.

Environmental Toxins

We are awash in a sea of exogenous estrogens, which just means anything that comes from outside the human body. Exogenous estrogens are chemicals in the environment that mimic the actions of estrogen in the body. These endocrine-disrupting compounds are often referred to as persistent organic pollutants (POPs). They include things like pesticides, plasticizers and industrial chemicals.

Some of these environmental hormones even come from our food and water. Milk is a major source of bovine (cow) estrogen and progesterone, and the global use of contraceptive pills may have made our water a source too. This is because women ingest the pills and then trace amounts of estrogen are urinated out. This is not completely removed by water treatment facilities, so it may end up in the water supply. The impact of this widespread estrogen in our environment is unknown, but it certainly can impact individuals who are most sensitive.

These estrogens have all kinds of consequences. Some can directly mimic estrogen, making your body think it has far too much of it. Others affect the estrogen receptors on your cells, blocking them so your real estrogen can't do its job. When this happens, you can enter a state called estrogen resistance. Since some cells can't hear the message estrogen is trying to send, and others hear the message too loudly, your body's own hormonal regulation gets confused and disrupted.

Because your tissues can't hear the messages estrogen is trying to send, your body may begin to produce more and more of it. The usual outcome is that progesterone levels fall even further and take a back seat to estrogen effects. At this point you enter a state of estrogen dominance, which can set off a cascade of hormonal imbalances.

As estrogen increases, progesterone may start to plummet further. Testosterone gets in on the action as well, often becoming relatively higher compared to progesterone and estrogen than it should be. This is when women start looking more like men, and you see patterns of male fat distribution (more fat around the belly) and hair growth (as can be the case with PCOS).

The symptoms of estrogen dominance vary from woman to woman, but they include:

- ✓ Overproduction of uterine lining tissue
- ✓ Heavy periods
- ✓ Fibroids
- ✓ Endometriosis
- ✓ PCOS
- ✓ Pronounced hip, butt, and thigh tissue
- ✓ Being overly stressed out
- ✓ Anxiety and/or depression

Basically, what you end up with is a dysregulation of the hormonal symphony, with all kinds of bad downstream consequences. How do you get estrogen back into balance? Well, this program will take you a long way toward getting this balance.

NORMAL MENSTRUAL CYCLE—PROGESTERONE DEFICIENT

Whereas estrogen is a growth promoter, progesterone is a growth trimmer. If estrogen and progesterone were landscapers, estrogen would grow the hedges and weeds and progesterone would trim the hedges and weed the garden. Estrogen and progesterone work together to keep the female physique lean and toned. Both hormones work together to keep fat from accumulating around the middle of the body. But when progesterone levels fall this becomes much more difficult.

Progesterone interacts with receptors all over the body, including in the fat tissues, muscle cells, brain, ovaries, uterus and breasts. So long as progesterone is in the Goldilocks zone, everything works beautifully. But when progesterone drops too low it can lead to issues.

When a hormone like progesterone declines, it impacts other hormones as well. For example, progesterone levels prime your tissues for other hormones to act—hormones like estrogen and thyroid. This means that when progesterone levels decline, these other hormones are negatively impacted as well.

As a result, you may experience hypothyroid-like symptoms. These include cold intolerance, constipation, hair loss, decreased quality of skin and nails, thinning of the eyebrows, depression, fatigue, slow thinking and memory issues. What this means for you is you may have periods of time where you feel tired, lethargic and sluggish and other times where you feel wired, anxious and buzzing inside.

Another area progesterone is crucial for is your brain and mood. Normal progesterone levels help maintain good levels of the GABA, the number one relaxing brain chemical that calms you and helps you get to sleep. Low progesterone can cause GABA levels to fall, spiking anxiety and causing insomnia. The outcome of all of this is that you may be feeling confused and frustrated as to why things just seem slightly off. You may even experience ovarian cysts, irregular menses, and unpredictable menstrual symptoms, and not have an explanation as to why.

You probably also notice a more difficult time keeping stomach fat at bay. Your body may feel more flabby and less toned. And the shape of your body may start to resemble something you no longer recognize.

The good news is that I can help you with these problems.

NORMAL MENSTRUAL CYCLE—ESTROGEN AND PROGESTERONE DEFICIENT

If you are estrogen and progesterone deficient, you have entered a state I refer to as "ovarian burnout." Whether by choice or circumstance your metabolic system is hyperactive, and as a result has depleted the strength of both estrogen and progesterone. This often happens after a period of extreme stress, illness, dieting or over-exercising.

That could be the cause, but just as often, the stress is more silent and sneaks up on you without you realizing. Typically, when this happens progesterone falls first, but if the stress continues, both hormones end up in a depressed flat line.

The female metabolism is very sensitive to stress. Too much stress to the female metabolism signals that it's not a good time to try to get pregnant. As a result, your metabolism becomes indifferent and uninterested.

This is much like what ovarian burnout feels like as well. It feels like some days you just want to lie in bed and do nothing, or stare at the wall and veg. Being indifferent and having no energy feels like life just isn't as exciting or enjoyable as it once was. Lack of estrogen and progesterone can cause these feelings.

It can also lead to fat gain and difficulty burning fat. Without progesterone's cortisol-blocking effects, you may see a redistribution of fat around your waist even if your weight does not change. This problem is compounded when you have a lack of estrogen since that hormone balances both the effects of cortisol and insulin.

Some women also experience hypothyroid-like symptoms when they are both estrogen and progesterone deficient. This is because both hormones influence thyroid. As a result, you may be feeling tired but at the same time wired, with a lack of interest in things you used to love. You may feel you just don't have the energy or drive to do much at all. You may even lose interest in sex too.

What this means is that you will likely have short stints of feeling energetic, motivated and focused, but more times than not you will feel tired and wired with anxious buzzing inside. But we can resolve those problems and rebalance your hormones, and this is precisely what you will learn to do in the next few chapters.

CAN YOUNG WOMEN BE IN MENOPAUSE?

Interestingly, younger women under extreme stress can actually enter a menopause-like state.

Stress impacts the hypothalamus and pituitary ovarian axis of women. When stress is extreme or prolonged the first effect is that progesterone falls. If the stress continues, estrogen levels fall as well. This is almost like self-induced menopause, since the changes are very similar.

This is essentially what happens in the athlete triad and PCOS to some degree.

If this describes you, see the section on The Metabolically Challenged Woman (below).

PERIMENOPAUSE—ESTROGEN HIGH OR FLUCTUATING AND PROGESTERONE DEFICIENT

What begins to happen when you move into perimenopause (the time just before you are in full-blown menopause) is that you have times when ovulation does not occur. This happens, in part, because you get improper amounts of FSH and LH to help the follicle grow and mature. The outcome is that the follicle won't rupture. It also happens as the number of viable eggs become diminished. This means no egg (thus no ovulation), but it also means you don't get the corpus luteum.

Remember that the corpus luteum is the source of progesterone, so if it isn't there, your progesterone levels plummet. This can lead to extended periods of estrogen exposure without progesterone to balance it out. Sometimes estrogen will be dominant and take over the show. At other times it will become completely wiped out since it is never getting any help from progesterone. This is one of the reasons perimenopause feels so unpredictable, uneasy, unbalanced even bipolar.

Under normal circumstances, estrogen and progesterone work together. Estrogen causes fat storage around the hips, butt, breast and thighs, and when acting with progesterone, keeps fat from being stored around the middle of the body. Both hormones also interact with receptors all over the body including in the fat tissues, muscle cells, brain, ovaries, uterus and breasts.

When estrogen and progesterone are working together in harmony, they are responsible for that beautiful hourglass shape that is the hallmark of the gorgeous female body. But when progesterone is no longer exerting influence, and estrogen is forced to do all the work itself, its levels will rise and fall unpredictably.

When estrogen is high sometimes and low other times, the tissues it signals become irregular in their function too. One minute the tissues and cells of the body see high estrogen and the next they see low. Rarely do they see normal levels. This is not a good outcome for the metabolism.

My point is that perimenopause can feel incredibly random, and it can drive your metabolism and your mind crazy as you try to keep up. As a result, you may be feeling motivated and clear one second, wired and anxious the next and depressed the next. No two days will feel exactly the same. You can feel like you are going a little crazy. This chart shows just how wild the estrogen rollercoaster ride can be during perimenopause:

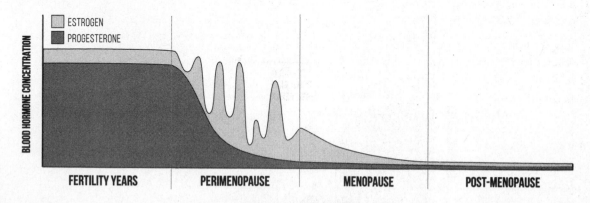

Your ovarian and uterine tissue are not getting the proper signals and rhythms anymore. Your periods will become irregular, unpredictable, lighter in flow and fewer in frequency. You may notice your eating habits change as well. While they may have been easier to maintain before, now it may be extremely difficult to manage unpredictable cravings and hunger that can range from ravenous to zero appetite at all.

You may also notice other areas of the body start to fare worse than before. Unpredictable digestion can ensue. Foods you tolerated previously may now cause heartburn or gas. You may find your thyroid and adrenal glands also take a beating. You may begin to experience symptoms like bowel changes, cold intolerance, irritability, frustration fatigue at times and excess energy at other time. This is all mainly due to the volatile nature of your fluctuating hormones.

One of the most impacted areas is the brain. Fluctuating estrogen levels create an unstable influence on serotonin and dopamine, leading to lack of motivation (dopamine) and feelings of insecurity or depression (serotonin). At the same time, low progesterone levels lead to falling levels of GABA, the number one relaxing brain chemical in the body. This, along with your estrogen levels bouncing around like a Ping-Pong ball, make for increased risk of worry and midnight monkey-mind where you can't shut your brain off to go to sleep.

So, it is no wonder you are feeling so unstable, volatile and out of balance—your hormonal system is partly to blame. But the good news is that by managing the 4Ms in a way to accommodate for your fluctuating hormones, you can regain your energy, stabilize your mood, and even burn off the stubborn fat that piles up for many women during this period.

MENOPAUSE—ESTROGEN DEFICIENT AND PROGESTERONE DEFICIENT

As perimenopause progresses and you move into menopause, ovulation stops completely and estrogen starts to decline as well. This means that both estrogen and progesterone fall over the course of perimenopause and menopause. But that doesn't happen in a smooth downward slope.

Instead, there are long periods of time when you have more estrogen than progesterone. This is very different than what happens during the normal menstrual cycle where there's an estrogen dominant time and a progesterone dominant time. This results in a period during which you're at risk for becoming more estrogen dominant, since while both progesterone and estrogen are falling, progesterone is falling faster than estrogen, as this chart shows:

Because these key female hormones fall during this time, testosterone, insulin, and cortisol begin to have a greater impact since there is less progesterone and estrogen to buffer their effects.

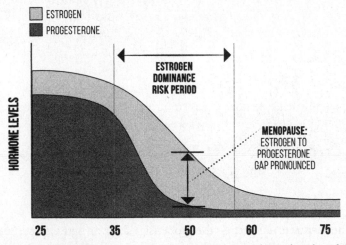

This is important. During menopause you end up in a situation where there's a decrease in estrogen, a decrease in progesterone, an increase in testosterone relative to these two hormones, and you become more stress-reactive and more insulin resistant. This is a perfect fat-gain formula. And it's why many women pack on the pounds—especially around the belly—during menopause.

To add insult to injury, your brain chemistry changes during this time as well. GABA, your major relaxing neurotransmitter, the brain-focusing chemical dopamine, and your self-esteem and relaxing neurotransmitter, serotonin, all decrease. One of the reasons this happens is because there are receptors for both estrogen and progesterone all over the body, including in your brain.

Fluctuations in estrogen and progesterone levels therefore impact brain chemistry, and this can lead to mood changes and cravings, making it even more difficult for women at menopause to maintain their weight.

POST-MENOPAUSE—ESTROGEN DEFICIENT AND PROGESTERONE DEFICIENT

After menopause is over and your cycle stops completely, you enter post-menopause. At this point, your metabolism looks more like a man's—you have higher testosterone relative to estrogen and progesterone. There are two likely outcomes at this point.

If you weren't able to manage your weight during menopause, you will end up with lots of extra fat—especially around the middle—and you'll have a harder time losing it, because you are no longer in a position to take advantage of your unique female fat-loss physiology. The other scenario is that you start looking like a man: you become more flat-chested and lose that hourglass shape.

The good news is that both of these situations can be managed by using the *Metabolic Renewal* program. If you learn to live, eat, and exercise in harmony with the hormonal changes you experience during and after menopause you can not only maintain your weight, but even burn fat.

I've seen it happen over and over again. I have seen hundreds (maybe thousands) of women go through this process, most with incredible results.

SPECIAL CASES

In addition to the various hormone types outlined above, this program can help you more effectively manage other special cases you may find yourself in. Pregnancy is a unique time in a woman's life where her metabolism acts slightly differently than it otherwise would. And some women don't have normal cycles, or suffer from other kinds of metabolic challenges. So let's look at some of these cases and how this program can help you.

PREGNANCY AND METABOLISM

Most women view pregnancy as a time where their metabolism abandons them in favor of their growing little one. They almost resign themselves to a ruined metabolism post-partum and start strategizing how to deal with this reality after they give birth.

Here's what most people don't know: pregnancy is one of the best things that can happen to a woman's metabolism. That is, if you do it right.

What Happens During Pregnancy?

If the egg is fertilized and implantation occurs, HCG levels will rise and keep the corpus luteum around long enough for the placenta to take over progesterone production. Interestingly, HCG is the first hormone of pregnancy and is used clinically to diagnose pregnancy. After about 8 weeks, the corpus luteum degrades and HCG levels fall off as the placenta takes on full-time duties of keeping estrogen and progesterone around.

Pregnancy is a unique time since it is one of the few times in a woman's life that she remains progesterone dominant. The only other times are during the second half of the menstrual cycle and when a woman is breastfeeding. Pregnancy through breastfeeding is certainly the most extended period of progesterone dominance a woman experiences.

This has many implications, one of which is to increase glucose intolerance and promote insulin resistance. Remember, estrogen makes women more insulin sensitive, so when it is suppressed for any length of time, insulin resistance can result. This sounds bad, but remember that an insulin-resistant and glucose-intolerant metabolism means more food for the growing baby.

Of course, many doctors and health coaches completely get this wrong. The old advice of telling women to "eat for two" is very stupid. There is no need to do this at all. In fact, if you want to heal your metabolism and be better off after pregnancy than before, you will not follow this bad advice.

Your body is intelligent and will increase your hunger as needed without your conscious effort. By consciously going into pregnancy thinking you now have a license to eat as much and whatever you want, you turn a great metabolic opportunity into a disaster.

It is estimated that a growing baby only requires about an extra 300 (second trimester) to 500 (third trimester) calories per day. There is no extra caloric requirement for the first trimester. There is no real need to count these calories, as your body will naturally and gently increase its SHMEC (sleep, hunger, mood, energy and craving) signals, allowing you to adjust your intake without much thought.

Studies show that more than half of pregnant moms gain more weight than is required for their pregnancy and subject themselves to metabolic issues like gestational diabetes along the way. Most expert resources give the following guidelines related to pregnancy weight gain.

- ✓ **Underweight pre-pregnancy** - BMI of less than 18.5 should gain 28-40 pounds
- ✓ **Normal weight pre-pregnancy** - BMI of 18.5-24.9 should gain 25-35 pounds
- ✓ **Overweight pre-pregnancy** - BMI of more than 25 should gain 15-25 pounds

The idea is to let the baby gain most of the weight while the mother adds enough fat and resources to sustain long-term breastfeeding. It is the combination of enough but not too much fat gain with breastfeeding that is such a powerful metabolic reset for women.

I will provide specific guidelines on how to eat and exercise if you are pregnant in Chapters 6 to 8. The key thing to understand for now is that pregnancy is not a metabolic disaster. At least, it doesn't have to be as long as you follow the *Metabolic Renewal* plan.

In fact, pregnancy can be a powerful metabolic reset, especially for women who breastfeed. First, it allows the woman to relax and recover. In fact, this is one of the only times relaxation and recovery are encouraged over the celebrated "stay busy and active" mindset of the Western world. Second, the progesterone dominance that persists through pregnancy and breastfeeding allows the body to be in more of an "eat more, exercise less" state without accumulating body fat, since the extra calories are being used for the baby.

Breastfeeding

Assuming you follow an intelligent diet and exercise plan (like the one outlined in this program) you will supply your baby with all it requires, and you will set the stage for a metabolic reset once the baby is born.

It is important to understand two points here. First, this metabolic reset is contingent on breastfeeding for at least six months, but longer is probably better—9 to 24 months may be optimal. Next, breastfeeding will slow fat loss in the short term but significantly accelerate fat loss later.

Research tells us that women who choose to bottle feed end up losing weight a little faster than their breastfeeding counterparts, but after about three months they are quickly surpassed by the breastfeeding moms. Most importantly, breastfeeders are shown to have leaner bodies—especially bellies and thighs—at all points after about six months. And those changes last.[10,11]

One of the reasons for this has to do with changes your body goes through when you first start breastfeeding. Lactation requires your caloric intake to remain a little higher than it would be if you weren't breastfeeding. Again, there is no reason to count calories, your SHMEC will lead you.

During this time, the insulin resistance and glucose intolerance experienced during pregnancy reduces, but prolactin levels rise, and this hormone can slow fat release down a bit while lactating. All of this is beneficial and healing to the metabolism if you give it time and patience, and you eat, exercise and live in a way that makes sense for what your body and your hormones are going through. This program will help you do that.

THE METABOLICALLY CHALLENGED FEMALE

What if you are one of the many women who do not follow the normal arc of menstruation, pregnancy and menopause? What if you don't menstruate normally and haven't in some time?

Perhaps you have polycystic ovarian syndrome (PCOS)—where your metabolism responds with a heightened stress response leading to insulin resistance, estrogen dominance, testosterone excess and fertility issues. Maybe you suffer from the athlete triad—a state where the stress from exercise shuts down your production of estrogen and progesterone. Or you might suffer from some other condition that impacts your cycle.

What do you do then?

The good news is that I have a program that will help you too. It may not return you to normal menstruation, but it will help you achieve and maintain your body shape and fat-loss goals. In my experience, the key to conditions like these is the hypothalamus and the pituitary gland—the areas in the brain that are the command and control center for your metabolism.

Your hypothalamus reads all the signals inside your body (from your thyroid, adrenals, ovaries and more) and outside your body (temperature, exercise, emotional stress, diet quality and quantity), integrates this information, and sends messages to your body on the proper way to respond. This hypothalamus connection to the rest of the metabolism is known as the hypothalamus-pituitary axis or the HPA. It is sort of like the information highway for your entire body.

There are three major parts to it: the HPT (hypothalamus pituitary thyroid axis), HPA (hypothalamus pituitary adrenal axis) and the HPG (hypothalamus pituitary gonadal axis—this includes your ovaries and testes). The HPA system is like a highly sensitive thermostat. When the body encounters metabolic extremes through illness, injury or stress this system reacts, creating metabolic dysfunction and damage.

Most of the women I have seen who are metabolically challenged suffer from imbalances in the HPA, whether it is due to PCOS, the athlete triad or some other condition. Typically, when you focus on rebalancing the HPA, the problem disappears.

That is precisely what this program is designed to do.

I can't promise to treat each and every case in this program. But I can tell you that *Metabolic Renewal* is specifically designed to help you rehabilitate your metabolism. So if you are metabolically challenged and suffer from one of the issues above (or others), this program is one of the best things you can do to heal.

I know that was a lot of scientific details and you didn't get this program to read a medical textbook. But hopefully you got a lot of education along the way about how your menstrual cycle works and how it influences your hormones.

How do you leverage this information to burn fat? How can you take what you learned here and create a program that fits your unique hormone type? The remainder of this program is designed to help you do just that.

WHAT YOU LEARNED IN THIS CHAPTER:

- ✓ The regularly menstruating woman has two phases to her cycle, each of which is predominated by either estrogen or progesterone.
- ✓ Eating and exercising in a way that honors this cyclic fluctuation of hormones can dramatically increase your fat-burning potential.
- ✓ Because each woman is different, each has a different hormone type. In some cases estrogen may be dominant, in others it may be deficient. In still others progesterone may be deficient.
- ✓ These different hormone types further influence a woman's ability to burn fat and overall health.
- ✓ As a woman approaches menopause first progesterone and then estrogen fall off. This leads to many different symptoms, including weight gain in some cases.
- ✓ When menopause occurs and the cycle stops completely, estrogen and progesterone are both depressed, and there is a relative increase testosterone.
- ✓ As a woman enters post-menopause, her metabolism looks more like a man's.
- ✓ Honoring this change in your hormones with diet, exercise and lifestyle changes can make all the difference in maintaining your hourglass shape and burning fat.
- ✓ Pregnancy is not a time to stop exercising and eat for two. In fact, it can be a time of metabolic reset, when approached correctly.
- ✓ Metabolically challenged women typically have imbalances in HPA. When you address these imbalances, the problem often resolves itself.

REDEFINING THE METABOLISM AND THE 4 METABOLIC TOGGLES

Distinctions matter, and when it comes to your metabolism, you have been given the wrong framework in which to understand it. This is why, before we go any further, I need to redefine metabolism for you.

Your metabolism is nothing but one big stress barometer. Its primary job is to register what is going on in the outside world, translate that information, and then tell your cells how to respond.

Obviously, your metabolism is registering all kinds of things, but two of the biggest influencers are eating and exercising. The energy you take in through food, combined with the energy you exert through exercise, can push metabolism into or out of balance.

Think of this like jumping from one end of a stream to another. If the gap is narrow, you can step over comfortably. If the gap is too wide, you are likely to land face down in the mud.

The trick to keeping your metabolism happy is making sure that the gap between energy intake and output remains narrow most of the time. If the gap widens on occasion, or for short periods of time, it's no big deal for the metabolism. But do this too often and that little stream will turn into a raging river with Class 5 rapids you can never get under control.

This is why you need to understand the four different ways you can manipulate energy intake and output. I call these "the 4 metabolic toggles" and you need to understand how they work so your eating and exercising make more sense from here on out.

THE 4 METABOLIC TOGGLES

The way you are used to thinking about weight loss is a battle between eating more and exercising less (EMEL) and eating less and exercising more (ELEM).

EMEL is the couch potato who sits around watching TV all day freebasing Doritos and crushing cokes. ELEM is the dieter who eats salads non-stop and runs around exercising all day like a chicken on speed.

The truth is these two metabolic states are not unique to the modern era. Your distant female hunter-gatherer ancestors encountered times where they definitely overate and sat around. They also had times where food was scarce, and they had to move a ton to find it.

The eat more, exercise less (EMEL) times probably came in a narrow window of time during late summer and early fall when fruits were abundant and easily harvested, and animals were slower, fatter and easier to catch as they prepared for winter.

The eat less, exercise more (ELEM) situation likely manifested in late winter and early spring when the weather was warming up but food and animals were harder to find.

There were two other metabolic states that were likely more prevalent to your ancient female metabolism, but you hear about them almost nowhere in the modern exercise and nutrition literature. The eat less, exercise less state (ELEL) and the eat more, exercise more condition (EMEM).

During most of the spring and summer your female ancestors would have been eating plenty and working plenty too (EMEM). During the late fall and most of winter, they would have been eating less and conserving the energy they expended (ELEL).

I don't want to bore you with an anthropological history lesson, but this insight is incredibly important for you to understand. What it tells you is that your metabolism is a flexible, adaptable system. If you want it to stay flexible and responsive, the last thing you want to do is try to subject it to a single metabolic state forever.

And that is exactly what the health and fitness world has been telling you to do. They want you to eat less and exercise more (ELEM) and they want you to try to live in this state forever. This is very bad advice, because eating less and exercising more is not something any female in the history of womankind would voluntarily do.

If your female ancestors were forced to be in an eat less, exercise more (ELEM) state for very long, it would have been a very stressful time. As a way to compensate, their metabolisms would have induced strong hunger and craving responses, and it would become more rigid by slowing metabolic rate and increasing metabolic efficiency to absorb more calories and expend less.

In other words, eating less and exercising more (ELEM) is not something the metabolism likes to do for too long. That metabolic outcome signals starvation, and results in extreme binge eating behavior. As soon as the situation is corrected (i.e., when food is readily available) it also triggers a wild swing back to eating more and moving less (EMEL).

It is important for you to understand that the advice to eat less and exercise more (ELEM) is actually priming your metabolism to get fat. Staying in this metabolic state more than a few weeks or months is convincing the metabolism it should start eating more and moving less as soon as possible.

This was a reasonable protective response for the realities of your ancient sisters: It kept them from starving to death. In today's world of fattening fast food, sugar-laced mocha lattes and all-you-can-eat buffets, it has become an unmitigated disaster. It would have been rare and unlikely for your ancestors to eat more than a few thousand calories in a day. Today it is not only possible but easy to consume 2,000 to 4,000 calories in just one meal.

What was once a genius adaptation primed by evolution for thousands of years has become a metabolic catastrophe.

Modern day research has now proven that dieting for long periods of time, using the eat-less-and-exercise more approach (ELEM), may be one of the primary causes of getting fat. The metabolism sees the wide gap of energy intake compared to output and decides that it better make adjustments for the future and push the energy gap back the other way to just as extreme an extent. It's trying to protect you. It registers all of this as a stress and thinks you are starving.

Have you ever wondered why the couch potato and the dieter both struggle with increased hunger, elevated cravings and unpredictable, unstable energy? It's because that is what a stressed out metabolism does. SHMEC goes out of check, and that is the last thing you want to have happen if you hope to make a sustainable lifestyle change.

To get sustainable and lasting results out of your metabolism, you want to stop Ping-Ponging back and forth between ELEM and EMEL and instead move to an ELEL and EMEM strategy.

ELEL is a lot like Europeans of the last century. They ate just a little, they moved a lot, and they exercised sparingly, if at all. This is a very relaxed, non-stressful, and healthy lifestyle. The calorie deficit created is more narrow and easily managed by the metabolism. You can live in the ELEL state for a long time.

EMEM is equivalent to the modern-day athlete. No athlete in her right mind cuts calories while trying to excel in her sport. And isn't the lean, tight and toned athlete the most sought after body type? EMEM, like ELEL, is far more balancing and sustainable for the metabolism.

Understanding these four different metabolic toggles gives you the tools required to escape the dieting mentality and the miserable consequences of dieting. The idea is to live most of your life cycling back and forth between ELEL and EMEM and only every so often move to EMEL or ELEM.

HOW IT WORKS IN THE REAL WORLD

Let me give you an example of how this works. Imagine a busy executive who travels most of the week, is home on the weekends and then takes the occasional vacation and holiday. She might choose to use an ELEL approach Monday through Thursday, because she is busy and has difficulty getting to the gym.

Friday through Sunday she lives more of an EMEM lifestyle since she is not working, can hit the gym, and likely eats and drinks a little more when she is socializing with friends and family.

She takes two or three vacations a year that last between one and two weeks. During this time she follows an ELEM approach, because she loves to hike, bike, climb and stay very active and does not think much about food. Since this is only for a week or two, the metabolism not only handles this but actually benefits from this approach.

When she goes up north for her holidays she follows more of an EMEL approach since the weather is cold, she is away from her gym, and she wants to eat and enjoy time with her family. Again, because this is only for a few weeks at most, the metabolism can use this time as a healing and restorative time.

Following a cyclical approach like this makes sense, is more intuitive and in line with her lifestyle, and far more beneficial to her health and fitness goals.

There are other ways to do it of course. Many young women who menstruate normally can adjust the toggles according to their cycle. During the follicular phase of the menstrual cycle (the two weeks after menses begins) when estrogen is higher, the body can tolerate more food and more exercise. EMEM works great to help maintain tight, lean tissue and perhaps lose some fat.

The luteal phase, the two weeks preceding menses when estrogen and progesterone are high together and progesterone dominates, is a great time for ELEL. Toward the end of the luteal phase, the body is more insulin-resistant and more stress-sensitive. ELEL works wonderfully here.

There are many different ways to approach this. The main point is to realize that your metabolism gets stressed very easily when energy intake and energy output are more extreme. By matching intake and output more closely you can create a sustainable and more enjoyable lifestyle.

STRUCTURED FLEXIBILITY

Now that you understand how the different metabolic toggles work, and you understand the idea of cycling, you will better understand how to apply the different toggles in the real world. But don't worry, I'm going to give you some more guidance in the next chapter on how to apply all of this in your own life to give yourself even more of a metabolic advantage.

What I want you to realize is that following a one-size-fit-all diet and exercise program does not and cannot work. The major goal of this program is to teach you how to be a metabolic detective, not a dieter.

To help you accomplish this I am going to give you a structure to begin with. Your job is to be flexible within that structure to create the perfect diet and lifestyle that works for you. I call this "structured flexibility," and it is the way you will work this process. It is the equivalent of teaching you to fish versus just giving you a fish.

To make it easier for you, I am going to provide a structure to follow in the beginning. You can think of this structure just like training wheels on a bike. You are not meant to follow this structure forever. Instead, you will use the structure only as a blueprint and beginning point. From there, your job is to begin to tweak, adjust and mold it to fit your unique metabolism, psychology and personal preferences.

Now that you understand the basics we can get into giving you a little more structure.

I want to leave you with one last important message: do not do the same thing everyone else does and think you have to follow things to the letter. I not only expect you to adjust things to fit your needs., I want you to.

WHAT YOU LEARNED IN THIS CHAPTER:

- ✓ Your metabolism is a stress barometer. Its job is to take information from the outside world and translate that into how your cells respond.
- ✓ Eating and exercising are two of the major inputs your metabolism reads.
- ✓ There are four metabolic toggles you can pull to shift your metabolism around.
- ✓ Most people are stuck in the battle between eat less and exercise more (ELEM) and eat more and exercise less (EMEL).
- ✓ There are two other toggles that are more efficient: eat less, exercise less (ELEL) and eat more exercise more (EMEM).
- ✓ You don't want to do any one thing for too long or your metabolism will adapt.
- ✓ The most important thing you can learn from this program is how to become a metabolic detective and create a plan that works for you.

MEALS

start with diet, because, frankly, it's more important than exercise.

If you only follow the exercise plan in this program you may get some results. But if you follow the diet and lifestyle portions, I guarantee you'll get results. And when you follow the full 4M framework, those results will come faster than you thought possible, and stick for good.

There is an old saying from bodybuilding circles that you can't out train a bad diet. Truer words have rarely been spoken. I don't care how hard you work out, if you're living on doughnuts, hot dogs, soda pop and pizza, you are not going to be healthy, and you are not going to lose weight.

However, finding the right diet for you can be tricky. We are each unique metabolically, psychologically and in our personal preferences. This means it's a fallacy that every person should eat the same diet.

As we have discussed throughout this program, you need to eat in a way that matches your hormone type. Your menstrual cycle, your time of life, and other factors can impact how you should eat.

Do you remember the Goldilocks effect? Well, diet is another place where this idea is important. You want to find the diet that is just right for you. Doing that largely comes down to carb balance.

This is not because carbohydrates are some evil junk food, like you've been told, but rather because they are powerful movers of metabolism both for better and for worse. Too much and you raise insulin levels, which makes it more likely that you will be in caloric excess, making it more likely those extra calories get stored as fat rather than muscle. Too little and you may induce your body's deprivation signals, raising cortisol and cravings while slowing your metabolic rate.

One of the best things you can do is find the right type, amount and timing of carbs for your body. I call this the "carbohydrate tipping point." It is the amount that is enough to keep SHMEC in check without going too far and causing excess calorie intake and insulin production.

I will teach you how to do that in this program. In fact, the entire program is designed to help you, as an individual, discover what works to optimize your metabolism.

To help you dial in your diet to your personalized needs, you'll take 3 steps:

✓ **Step 1 – Start with the Base Meals Plan:** First, I am going to introduce you to the core dietary plan that I start everyone on. This is your starting point, and it's the place you come back to if you ever get confused about what to eat or if you stop getting the results you want.

✓ **Step 2 – Modify Based on Your Hormone Type:** Next I am going to teach you how to modify this diet based on your hormone type or if you are in a special case scenario like those we discussed in Chapter 4.

✓ **Step 3 – Customize Based on Your Unique Metabolism:** Finally, I will teach you how to take all of this further and personalize the program for your specific metabolism.

Let's get started.

THE *METABOLIC RENEWAL* BASE MEALS PLAN

The starting point for all of the diet variations in this plan is what I call The 3-2-1 Diet. This is the ELEL approach.

✓ 3 meals
✓ 2 of those meals have protein and veggies only (a little fruit is allowed)—alternatively, these meals can be shakes
✓ 1 of those meals contains a small portion of starch

Simple, right?

There is no calorie counting on this program. You will know you are in a caloric deficit if you are burning fat and you are moving toward that hourglass shape, regardless of your age or current body shape.

As you will learn in your *Metabolic Renewal Transformation Tracker*, the easiest way to know whether this is happening is by measuring, which I strongly encourage you to do weekly. Taking those measurements provides a steady stream of motivating feedback to keep you going.

Portion control is important, but easily managed by eating more foods with the right levels of water, fiber and protein. You don't need special containers or a food scale.

When it comes to your first two meals of the day, I don't want to be too dogmatic about protein and veggies only. Some fruit

QUALITY COUNTS TOO

The quality of your food is also crucial to your health and weight loss efforts. Pesticides and other non-organic compounds can have hormone-like effects that wreak havoc on your metabolism. Most of the protein we get in the supermarket comes from what's called factory farms, or CAFOs. These animals are fed a diet they were never meant to eat, not to mention exposed to extraordinary amounts of antibiotics and other chemicals meant to keep them "healthy" in the rather criminal conditions in which they live.

As often as your budget allows, choose organic produce and pasture-raised, grass-finished meat products. It's good for you and good for the environment.

is allowed too. What you need to understand here is the framework. Start thinking about protein and veggies as the core of your diet.

The easiest way to think about it is this: put veggies on three-quarters of your plate and protein on one quarter.

Of course, these meals can also be healthy shakes if you prefer. Whole foods are typically better for the metabolism, but shakes offer a quick and healthy alternative for many time-strapped people. You will see that they are featured prominently in the *12-Week Metabolic Renewal Meal Plan*, where you will find many healthy and delicious options.

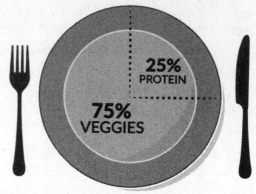

For the last meal of the day—your meal with starch—the easiest way to think it is as follows:

Take half of your plate and fill it with veggies. Then place a small piece of protein on about a quarter of it, and add a small portion of starch to the other quarter.

Again, you don't have to be dogmatic about it. You could have a shake here too, but most people want to eat a meal at dinner time.

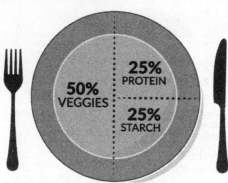

When it comes to starch portion, it is best if you eat starches naturally rich in water compared to those that are more dry. This means tubers, squashes, beans, rice and oats. These foods will be better choices compared to the drier starches like breads and cereals. Of course, the refined junk food stuff should be avoided, except on rare occasions.

Which veggies should you choose? What forms of protein? How do you know which foods to focus on and which to avoid? This is all spelled out in the "Roll Your Own Meal Plans" section of the *12-Week Metabolic Renewal Meal Plan*.

Or you can make all of this even easier on yourself and follow the actual menus and recipes in the meal plan. They were specifically designed to go with this program and include mouthwatering recipes like Coconut Herbed Frittata and Savory Steak with Mushrooms.

Remember, this 3-2-1 Diet is the basic meal plan you can always return to if you get lost, don't get the results you want, or are otherwise confused.

But if you want to take full advantage of your female fat-burning potential, you will fine-tune this diet as follows.

MEAL MODIFICATIONS FOR MENSTRUATING WOMEN

All menstruating women—regardless of their hormone type—can take The 3-2-1 Diet and modify it as follows.

During the first two weeks of your cycle (the follicular phase), you can add one additional meal of protein, veggies and starch. As you'll learn in the next chapter, you can also exercise a little more in this part of your cycle. This is an EMEM approach.

Why would you want to add a meal and additional exercise during the follicular phase of your cycle?

The follicular phase is a time of estrogen dominance, which makes the body more insulin-sensitive. This means it will store less fat in a calorie surplus, opting to gain lean muscle instead. It will also burn less muscle in a calorie deficit leaning towards fat loss instead.

Remember that a lean, fit and healthy female body has tight toned muscle and a lean midsection. That is precisely the body type that cycling your diet this way will help you achieve.

The menus in your *12-Week Metabolic Renewal Meal Plan* offer an optional additional meal for women in the follicular phase of their cycle. You can add this meal, or you can simply create an additional "roll your own" meal during your day.

During the last two weeks of your cycle—the luteal phase—you will dial back your exercise a bit (details to follow in chapter 8), and you will stick to The 3-2-1 Diet.

This is an eat less, exercise less approach (ELEL), and you want to do this in your luteal phase because at this point progesterone dominates making the body a little more insulin resistant.

Also, the week before menses can see sharp declines in both estrogen and progesterone leading to a more stress reactive physiology. Most women will do best with eating less and doing less stressful exercise during this time.

In the health and nutrition world, this pattern of eating is often referred to as "cycling," and it's especially powerful, because it works with the natural compensatory nature of the metabolism.

Remember, the metabolism is adaptive and reactive to everything. If you constantly use the same approach, it will react quickly and all fat-loss efforts will stall or reverse. Using the cycling approach allows you to change with your metabolism, working with it rather than against it.

Just cycle your diet along with your menstrual cycle, and you will kick your fat-burning furnaces into high gear.

Then you can add the following modifications based on your specific hormone type to take all of this a step further.

Normal Menstrual Cycle—Estrogen and Progesterone Balanced

If you fall into this hormone type, the thing you want to focus on is adjusting your diet as your estrogen and progesterone adjust. Your system is designed to have elevated estrogen during the first part of the cycle, and a progesterone-dominant time after ovulation.

When estrogen is elevated, the metabolism is building up its resources, allowing you to tolerate food better. When progesterone is high, it switches gears, encouraging you take it easy so you can support a potential child.

If you want to look good and feel great, simply duplicate this in your life. Cycle your diet so you are eating more and

WHAT IF YOU ARE ON BIRTH CONTROL OR HORMONE REPLACEMENT THERAPY?

If you are taking birth control or hormone replacement therapy, dietary cycling will still work. However, there are a couple of things to be aware of.

First, your metabolism will behave more like it does in the second half of your cycle.

This means you will be a little more stress reactive and carb sensitive.

So pay careful attention to your SHMEC, and your body composition goals. If your SHMEC goes out of check (learn more about this below), or if you aren't burning fat, go back to The 3-2-1 Diet, and work through the AIM protocol below to adjust this diet to your personal needs.

exercising more (EMEM) when estrogen is high, and relaxing and being more careful with your diet and exercise (ELEL) when progesterone takes over.

You are also going to want to make one big change, if possible, that will help rebalance your insulin levels. Women are more insulin resistant during the second half of their cycle. To adjust for that, you can:

✓ Count up the amount of carbohydrate grams you eat per day; let's say it is 200g.
✓ Simply replace half of those carbohydrate grams with grams of protein during the second half of your cycle only. Whey protein is an especially good way to make this switch.

Now, I don't want you stressing about measuring everything precisely, as that's not practical, so instead, use this rule of thumb: Each bite of starch (about the size of a tablespoon) is around 10g of carbohydrate. So 100g of carbohydrate would be 10 bites of starch in a day.

This one change can immediately put you in a better nutritional state to work with the unique hormones in each the two parts of your menstrual cycle.

Normal Menstrual Cycle—Estrogen Dominant

Recall from our earlier discussion that estrogen causes fat storage around the hips, butt, breasts and thighs and, when acting normally, works with progesterone to keep fat from being stored around the middle of the body. When estrogen gets too high and starts to dominate, it can lead to issues.

WHY IS THIS DIET DIFFERENT THAN OUR OTHER PROGRAMS?

If you've purchased *The Metabolic Factor, Metabolic Aftershock, or Metabolic Prime,* you may wonder why this approach is different and how it fits with our other programs.

The truth is that it isn't all that different. It just looks that way on the surface.

Most people do not do well with too much carbohydrate.

But the idea that you should starve your body of carbs forever isn't right either. Your metabolism adapts and reacts, compensating for this reduction in carbohydrate.

The result?

Your metabolism can slow way down.

Cycling the diet prevents this.

The Metabolic Factor is our entry level program, and introduces you to cycling with what you can think of as mini-cycles. It cycles carbs every few days to keep the metabolism guessing.

Metabolic Aftershock and *Metabolic Prime* are both eat less, exercise less (ELEL) approaches that focus on the 3-2-1 Diet (we just didn't call it that) with an optional carb refeed thrown in.

If you've been following any of these program, moving in the direction outlined here will take your results to the next level and it will help you more effectively integrate this way of eating and living into your life.

Estrogen dominance can manifest in your metabolism as excesses in some places and deficiencies in others. For example, you may notice increased blood flow, cramping and clotting during menses (excess), but also lack of energy and mental depression at the same time (deficiency). You probably notice a thickening layer of fat, and a more stubborn area, around the hips, butt and thighs. Cellulite may be more pronounced as well.

This is all due to estrogen's impact on small cellular receptors called alpha receptors that slow fat release from certain areas of the body. The hips, butt and thighs are notorious for being rich in these alpha receptors.

So, you need to adjust to take in less estrogen, stop making as much estrogen in your own metabolism, and help your body eliminate estrogen. The body gets rid of extra estrogen by processing it in the liver and then kicking it out into the digestive tract via the gallbladder. From there, it latches onto fiber to be carried out of the body. Too little fiber hinders this flushing.

This is why you must focus on fiber, fiber and more fiber, along with water, water and more water, if you are estrogen dominant. Shoot for a minimum of 30g of fiber per day and really try to get closer to 100g. Be careful though—fiber needs to be added slowly into the diet to avoid digestive upset. Too much too quickly and you will have traffic overload.

To make this easier for you it might be helpful for you to know that a cup of vegetables contains about 8g of fiber. A piece of fruit contains about 3g of fiber. Although you can find other foods that contain more fiber, most of these also contain way more starch and sugar. It is always wise to get your fiber from vegetables first (they contain very little starch or sugar) and fruit next (they contain a lot of water).

There are some things about fiber you need to understand. There are foods that contain fiber but are also devoid of water and loaded with starches and sugar. These types of fibers include breads and are not what you want. To get all the benefits of fiber, without any downsides, stick with green vegetables and low-sugar fruits like berries, apples, pears and citrus.

One of the best ways to accomplish your fiber goals is to set the goal of having one large salad per day and one small salad before dinner each evening.

In addition to increasing your fiber intake, here are a couple of additional suggestions if you are estrogen dominant:

- ✓ High-fat foods concentrate hormones, so getting your fats from vegetable sources versus animal sources may help.
- ✓ Organic foods may also be a consideration. Non-organic foods are sprayed with chemicals that can work as estrogen mimics in the body. Eliminating these chemicals can help.

I know these things can be a little bit of a pain, and if you are not able to take these additional steps, just know that the extra fiber step is the most critical.

Normal Menstrual Cycle—Progesterone Deficient

You could easily call progesterone the stress barometer hormone. As stress levels rise, progesterone levels are the first to fall. So when it comes to meals, your goal is to help reduce or compensate for stress.

In terms of diet, you want to focus on what I call the "carbohydrate tipping point." A lot of people avoid carbohydrates because they have heard that they make you fat. This is not true. The trick is to get enough but not too much, and to eat them during times when they may have more benefit.

One of the reasons the body releases stress hormones is to help release stored sugar so it can be used. By giving your body more complex carbohydrates preemptively we can help reduce some stress.

Begin by having your carbohydrates in and around the times you feel most volatile and not at any other times. This will be most useful toward the end of the day.

Here's the rule I want you to follow, which I call the "Half-in-Half" Rule, which will easily begin to get you closer to a level of blood sugar that will be less stressful for you:

- ✓ I want you to consume half of the amount of carbohydrates you are currently eating, and only eat them in the second half of the day (after 3 p.m.), especially at night.
- ✓ If you are already cutting carbs (<100 g per day), then I want you to double the amount of carbs you are eating and eat them in the second half of the day (after 3 p.m.)

As mentioned before, there's no need for stressing about measuring everything precisely; just use this rule of thumb: Each bite of starch (about the size of a tablespoon) is around 10g of carbohydrate. So 100g of carbohydrate would be 10 bites of starch in a day.

Normal Menstrual Cycle—Estrogen and Progesterone Deficient

Estrogen and progesterone sensitize each other's hormone receptors. This means they are so interdependent that when one falls the other can act irregularly even if its levels are normal.

When these hormones fall, you can often feel mood issues that are best described as an anxious depression—always worried, with a racing mind, but unable to get anything done.

Here the rule I want you to follow—I call it the "Front Load, Back Load" Approach. This is a very simple way of giving you carbs when you most need them, at the beginning of the day (the first meal) and the end of the day (the last meal of the day):

- ✓ If you are currently eating 200 grams of carbohydrates a day, I want you to split those carbs up evenly between your first meal and last meal of the day (i.e., 100g in the morning and 100g in the evening).
- ✓ If you are carb restricting, then double the amount of carbs you are currently eating (up to 200g per day) and split them as outlined.

Again, I don't want you stressing about measuring everything precisely. Remember that each bite of starch (about the size of a tablespoon) is around 10 g of carbohydrate. So 100 g of carbohydrate would be 10 bites of starch in a day.

This approach will control high rises in stress hormones in the morning as well as keep them suppressed in the evening so you can sleep as well.

MEAL MODIFICATIONS FOR PERIMENOPAUSE, MENOPAUSE AND POST-MENOPAUSE

Perimenopause is a time when progesterone starts to drop off due to the fact that you are no longer ovulating regularly. As you progress into menopause, estrogen falls off as well, and eventually your period stops altogether. At this point you are in post-menopause.

Perimenopause and menopause are especially challenging times for women for many reasons. Many experience fat gain, especially around the belly, butt and thighs, and watch in horror as their beautiful hourglass shape disappears. Mood swings, cravings, brain fog and other symptoms that are a result of fluctuating hormone levels make things worse.

What do most women do to counteract this? They do what society tells them, and they eat less and exercise more (ELEM). Which is extremely unfortunate, because menopause is one of the worst times you can take this approach.

Why?

Your body is acutely sensitive to stress during this time. Eating less and exercising more (ELEM) is a stressor on the body. Cortisol goes up, and then you pack on fat for all of the reasons we discussed in Chapter 3.

In addition, many women become very carb sensitive during this time, and may even enter a state of insulin resistance due to their changing body chemistry. This means you have to carefully monitor your carb intake.

To account for all of this, the dietary plan I recommend for women during this time of life is a little different:

- ✓ Start with The 3-2-1 Diet.
- ✓ After that, the first thing you will want to do is add a snack. This strategic snack is important at this stage, because the menopausal metabolism is far more stress-reactive.

In fact, it is so stress-reactive that going longer than 4 hours without food can result in blood sugar changes and stress hormone elevations that throw SHMEC out of check (you'll learn more about SHMEC in the next chapter). This preemptive strategic snack helps blunts these effects beautifully.

Next, I recommend that you replace your morning veggie and protein meal with a shake. Whole foods are always preferred, but protein shakes provide a convenient and repeatable fuel source for women during this transition, which often comes with a feeling of being overwhelmed and doing too much.

Of course, this morning shake approach is a convenient option for younger women too, but it can be especially useful in menopausal changes.

You will find many delicious and filling shake recipes in your *12-Week Metabolic Renewal Meal Plan*. In fact, you will see that most of the menus include a shake for breakfast for everyone on the program.

My last recommendation for women in perimenopause, menopause and post-menopause is to make sure your starch meal is at night. The reason for this is that eating a little starch at night can help you sleep, and many women have problems with insomnia during this time of life.

The reason starch helps with sleep in many women is because at this stage of life blood sugar levels are less stable and may drop sooner and faster when skipping meals or foregoing starch.

What does the body do to combat this blood sugar effect? It releases stress hormones like adrenaline, which increase blood sugar and also turn on your monkey mind (that worrying part of your brain that won't shut up). These can both keep you up at night.

Having a little bit of starch preemptively at night can raise blood sugar enough to keep this effect from happening.

Now, don't worry, all of this is laid out in detail in your *12-Week Metabolic Renewal Meal Plan*. There are menus you can follow, options to help you roll your own meals, and simple tips on how to add snacks and starch to your program where necessary.

Perimenopause—Estrogen Fluctuating, Progesterone Deficient

The key to remember with perimenopause is that your two female hormones that are designed to work in tandem are upset by the deficient level of progesterone, with estrogen levels rising to compensate, then crashing when depleted.

Because of this estrogen rollercoaster, perimenopause can feel incredibly random in its effects, driving your metabolism and your mind crazy as you try to keep up. You may notice your eating habits—which may have been easier to maintain before—become extremely difficult to manage due to unpredictable craving and hunger that can range from ravenous to zero appetite at all.

Your entire system is forever losing its cyclical rhythm, meaning you are more sensitive to fat storage from food and more reactive to fat storage from stress. It's a double whammy.

You need to focus on fiber, protein and water. These foods fill you up quickly, keep you full for a longer time and balance blood sugar so you will have fewer cravings. To make this simple for you, think salads, soups, shakes and scrambles.

There is one other thing you can do that is super-powerful, and that is to use cocoa powder. Now remember, cocoa is different than chocolate. Chocolate is cocoa powder combined with fat and sugar. I am just talking about the cocoa powder. It contains serotonin and dopamine mimickers along with other compounds that relax and focus the mind by undoing some of the negative brain effects caused by fluctuating estrogen and low progesterone.

Take 1 tablespoon of cocoa powder and put it in a cup. Then gently pour hot water on top while stirring to avoid clumping. Drink this to avoid cravings and stabilize your volatile system. You can use this every day, multiple times per day. It works wonders.

Menopause—Estrogen and Progesterone Deficient

Estrogen and progesterone work together, aiding each other to keep fat from accumulating around the middle of the body. When progesterone and estrogen levels fall, this becomes much more difficult. This is why you may be dealing with the dreaded menopause belly. Your weight may not have changed, but your body shape definitely has changed.

Estrogen and progesterone also act to block the actions of the stress hormone cortisol. Take these hormones away and insulin levels and cortisol levels rise together along with a usual increase in calories due to cravings and hunger elevations. This is a deadly combination that can quickly lead to increased belly fat.

In terms of diet, your approach should be to use the "Front Load, Back Load" Approach. This gives you carbs when you most need them, at the beginning of the day (the first meal) and the end of the day (the last meal of the day):

- ✓ If you are currently eating 200 grams of carbohydrates a day, I want you to eat almost all of the carbs first thing in the morning, or the last thing at night.
- ✓ If you are carb restricting, then I want you to double your carbs (up to 200g per day) and then split them as outlined.

This approach will control high levels of stress hormones in the morning as well as keeping them suppressed in the evening so you can sleep as well.

As always, don't worry about measuring everything precisely, just use the rule of thumb that each bite of starch (about the size of a tablespoon) is around 10g of carbohydrate, so 100g of carbohydrate would be 10 bites of starch in a day.

Post-Menopause—Estrogen and Progesterone Deficient

Post-menopause can be particularly troubling for the female physique since testosterone, which is normally much lower than estrogen and progesterone before menopause, can, in some women, continue to be produced at its previous levels. This means that testosterone is relatively high compared to estrogen and progesterone—not a good hormonal combination for women.

This results in a metabolism that resembles more a man's than a woman's, resulting in a physique that takes on more male traits. Don't worry, life's fair: the reverse happens to men as they age. Their testosterone falls while estrogen levels rise and they become more like a woman than a man. I know, it sounds like a cruel joke of nature, right?

Due to the suppression of estrogen and progesterone and the relative increase in testosterone, insulin and cortisol levels typically rise during this time. This, along with a usual increase in calories due to cravings and hunger elevations, further contributes to postmenopausal belly fat. Your body may feel more flabby with less tone. Of course, there are the health issues too: thinning bones, increased risk of heart disease and cancer and more.

Due to the suppression of estrogen and progesterone, cortisol and insulin effects are amplified. Add to this the relative increase in testosterone and you have the perfect scenario for fat gain around the middle as well as elevated risk of heart-related conditions.

For meals, you must again focus on the carbohydrate tipping point. One of the reasons the body releases stress hormones is to help release stored sugar so it can be used. By giving your body more complex carbohydrates preemptively we can reduce some of this stress.

Complex carbohydrates are starch sources that provide long chains of starch, such as those found in potatoes, rice, beans, bread and pasta. Remember, eating enough of these foods, but not too much, allows you to control stress hormones and insulin while providing some enjoyability to the diet.

You should use the "Front Load, Back Load" Approach, giving you carbs when you most need them, at the beginning of the day (the first meal) and the end of the day (the last day of the meal.) So, if you are currently eating 200 grams of carbohydrates a day I want you to eat almost all of the carbs first thing in the morning and last thing at night. In other words, divide the amount of carbs you are eating between those two meals and try not to eat them anywhere else. This will control surges in stress hormones in the morning and suppress them in the evening so you can sleep.

MEAL MODIFICATIONS FOR SPECIAL CASES

Your hormone type isn't the only thing that impacts the diet you design for yourself. Some special metabolic cases can also influence your best course of action. Here is some dietary information specific to pregnant women and those who are metabolically challenged.

THE PREGNANT WOMAN

Most new research on pregnancy and exercise shows that we may have gotten a little too carried away with telling women to "take it easy," especially when that message is combined with "eat for two."

The real message should be to listen to your body, keep yourself healthy and happy, and support your growing baby. Then focus on body composition goals after you give birth. Doing things intelligently during pregnancy allows that process to be much easier.

Every woman will be different, but my clinical experience has been that women following The 3-2-1 Diet do wonderfully during pregnancy and after, as long as they keep a couple of things in mind.

First, when you are pregnant, you need to pay careful attention to your hunger signals and follow them. So you need to tune in to your SHMEC (sleep, hunger, mood, energy and cravings), and adjust your diet as necessary. I'll talk more about how to optimize your diet using SHMEC in the next chapter, but for women who are pregnant, the solution is simple:

Follow The 3-2-1 Diet, and eat more when you are hungry. You can add a snack. You can add a meal. You can even add a snack and a meal if your hunger dictates.

Your body will naturally indicate how many calories you need to consume to support your growing baby. How will it do this? By making you hungry. So, follow those hunger signals, and add snacks or meals as needed.

If you wish, you can follow the menus and recipes in your *12-Week Metabolic Meal Plan,* and add any meal or snack you wish as necessary. You can also simply "roll your own" meals and snacks if you like.

Breastfeeding Eating Style

After baby is born, things will change a little bit.

Research shows that the longer you breastfeed the healthier it is for your baby and future metabolism.[12] The longer a woman breastfeeds, the more insulin sensitive they become. Studies have shown that if you bottle feed, you may lose weight faster at first. But this slows down, and we know that most women lose more weight by breastfeeding longer.

You will want to start with the 3-2-1 Diet, and then begin cycling as described above after 4-8 weeks. Even if menstruating hasn't resumed, this is safe for you to do post-pregnancy. Your metabolism thrives on change, so use the cycling approach to work with it instead of against it and you'll find post-pregnancy can be a great time for a metabolic reset.

THE METABOLICALLY CHALLENGED WOMAN

Women who are metabolically challenged are those with a rigid, stubborn or inflexible metabolism. Usually this will manifest itself as some kind of "disease state"—PCOS, hypothyroidism, the athlete triad syndrome, adrenal fatigue and others.

The nutrition protocol is the same for all of them, because the root cause of all these issues is the same: namely an imbalance in the hypothalamus and the pituitary.

The downstream effects vary, but the way to bring this axis back online is to follow The 3-2-1 Diet, and then add a few supplements based on which condition you suffer from.

Remember, the HPA is the command and control center of the metabolism. This area is extremely sensitive and responsive to stressors. One of the major stressors to the metabolism is meals that come too frequently or infrequently. There is that Goldilocks effect again. The 3:2:1 approach strikes the perfect balance and has been proven in my clinic.

Here are the supplements I recommend for the main conditions I see women suffer from.

Hypothyroidism

Ashwagandha 500 to 1500mg per day. This herb helps thyroid hormone function better with the cells it interacts with. Ashwagandha also aids the hypothalamus and pituitary. It is best for those who feel what we call "wired but tired"—wired on the inside but physically tired in the body.

PCOS

Berberine 500 to 1500mg per day and alpha lipoic acid 200 to 600mg per day. Berberine has been shown in studies to outperform the insulin-sensitizing drug metformin specifically in those with PCOS.[13] Alpha lipoic acid works synergistically with berberine to help the liver and cells manage the effects of insulin issues.

Adrenal Fatigue

Rhodiola rosea 300 to 600mg per day. This is one of the best supplements I have found to restore balance to the HPA. Research has shown that it is an excellent aid to those dealing with fatigue due to overwork, overtraining or long periods of excess stress and strain.[14]

Athlete Triad

Rhodiola rosea 300 to 600mg per day and L-glutamine powder 5 to 15g per day. Rhodiola works on the HPA as noted above, while L-glutamine works on the 3-, 4- and 5-star generals of the metabolism: the immune system, muscles and the gut respectively. Glutamine is a key player in all these areas and can make a huge difference.

Menopause and menstrual issues

Vitex (chasteberry) 200 to 400mg per day. This herb acts on the hypothalamus to restore normal function of the HPA and it's signaling to the ovaries. In this way Vitex can deliver estrogen and progesterone balancing effects.

Look, I know this isn't as straightforward as some of the other dietary dogma that's out there. But the truth is rarely simple. The fact is that you need to learn how to eat and live in accord with your unique metabolism. You need to become a dietary detective. Which leads me to what I want to talk about in the next chapter.

WHAT YOU LEARNED IN THIS CHAPTER:

✓ Listening to your body, no matter what hormone type, is key to finding the best meal plan for you.

✓ The importance of SHMEC (sleep, hunger, mood, energy and cravings) at all times, especially when pregnant.

✓ Introduction of the base diet, called The 3-2-1 Diet, which will help to reset the metabolic cycle.

✓ Variations in dietary needs based on hormone type.

✓ The use of meal replacement shakes can be a benefit to resetting the metabolic rate for a busy lifestyle, but whole foods have the greatest positive impact.

✓ What supplements are best recommended for those who are metabolically challenged.

BECOME A METABOLIC DETECTIVE TO PINPOINT THE RIGHT DIET FOR YOU

This chapter is the most important one in the program for a very important reason: we want the changes you make to last a lifetime.

You have likely heard about the recent and now famous study of the biggest losers from the television series *The Biggest Loser*.[15] These contestants spent three months losing as much weight as possible under an extreme eat less, exercise more program (ELEM). They were then followed for six years after they left the show. What do you think they got for their efforts?

They regained almost all the weight and had lasting negative metabolic changes still impacting them six years later. Part of the reason for this was the extreme and wrong use of the eat less, exercise more approach (ELEM) to weight loss.

Another issue was the one-size-fits-all approach. You are not like every other woman on the planet. You are unique metabolically, psychologically and in your personal preferences. To be successful and make it stick, you must stop studying programs and diets and start studying yourself. This is the only way to know how eating carbohydrates affects you versus your girlfriend, mom or sister.

My goal is to give you the tools so that you will never, ever diet again. Instead, you will learn to view this as a journey where each step along the way teaches you more and more about your own needs and reactions, so that, in time, you know exactly what works and what does not for you.

Even after you create this unique approach for yourself, guess what? Metabolism is changing all the time, so you may need to periodically readjust. This is why learning to be a metabolic detective is so important. This is not about following a protocol, but instead about learning a process. Following a diet is like being given a fish. Learning to be a metabolic detective is teaching you to fish.

It's like my hero Bruce Lee says, "absorb what is useful, discard what is not, and add what is uniquely your own." This is what the metabolic detective process will teach you.

Start by choosing the diet program in Chapter 6 that matches your hormone type. If you follow it (as well as the exercise plan in the next chapter) as outlined for 7-14 days but don't start seeing changes, feel different, or your SHMEC is out of check, you may need to fine-tune your nutrition plan a little further for your personal needs. Here's how to do that.

KEEP YOUR SHMEC IN CHECK

As you know, SHMEC is an acronym that stands for sleep, hunger, mood, energy and cravings. During the first 7-14 days of this program you may notice fluctuations in these five parameters. This is normal as your metabolism adapts.

After 14 days, if you are experiencing any combinations of poor sleep, lots of hunger, unbalanced mood, unpredictable energy and/or increased cravings, this is a sign that your metabolic hormones have not adapted. At this point you will need to play detective a bit and begin tweaking and adjusting your approach. Here are some recommendations.

STEP #1: FEED THE LEAN

If you happen to be a lean, fit, athletic person already, it is possible that you may want to increase your starchy foods slightly to help maintain muscle. Being highly insulin sensitive gives you an advantage with these foods. With your metabolism, they are unlikely to lead to fat gain and more likely to result in muscle shaping.

If your SHMEC is not stable and you feel you could use the extra fuel, add a little bit of starch, first after your workout (e.g., ½ banana) and next at your dinner (e.g., a bit of sweet potato with your salmon and kale).

While many carbohydrates will work based on your tastes and needs, the four best and cleanest carbohydrates to consider are oats, potatoes, rice (especially brown rice) and sweet potatoes. Balanced with ample vegetable and protein intake they are uniquely suited to body change and resetting the body's dietary needs. Balancing this within your carbohydrate tipping point, based on your hormone type, allows you enough energy to get the job done without storing fat.

When thinking about amounts, think in bites. Three regular bites of a highly starchy food, each about the size of a tablespoon, will provide 15 grams or so of carbohydrates. So when adding in starches, add in 3 bites post workout (e.g., ½ banana), and 3 bites for dinner (e.g., 3 bites of a baked sweet potato). You can then slowly increase your starch intake by 3 bites (3 tablespoons or 15g) at a time at each of these times until your SHMEC is back in check.

Here are some options you can choose from for your post-workout or dinner-starch options.

Post-Workout

Best Options

- ½ cup of brown rice
- ½ cup oats

- ½ large sweet potato
- ½ potato

Additional Possibilities

- ½ banana added to your smoothie
- ½ cup quinoa

- 1 cup black beans
- 1 cup pumpkin or other starch

Dinner

- ½ cup brown rice
- ½ medium baked potato

- ½ medium sweet potato
- ½ cup quinoa

But what if you aren't a fit, athletic person or adding a little starch doesn't resolve imbalances in your SHMEC? It's time to move on to Step 2.

STEP #2: BECOME A DIET DETECTIVE AND FIND THE RIGHT DIET FOR YOU

There are two things required for sustained and lasting fat loss: hormonal balance and consuming fewer calories. You have learned that it is rarely, if ever, necessary to count calories. When you eat intelligently to balance hormones, the calories almost always take care of themselves by way of automatically reduced hunger.

Still, this can be a bit disconcerting to those so used to the dieting mentality. After all, you can count calories, which makes you feel like you are more in control. But how the heck do you get a quantitative assessment of what is going on with your hormones?

Well, now you know you can. It's called your SHMEC.

Remember, your sleep, hunger, mood, energy and cravings are biofeedback cues. Hormones impact these sensations either directly or indirectly. So by paying attention to how your body feels, you can understand whether your metabolism is balanced or not.

For the first 14 days your SHMEC may be out of check. That's normal. It takes some time for your body to adjust to this new way of eating and exercising. If, after 14 days on the program, your SHMEC is in check, then your metabolic hormones are in balance. If you are losing fat, then you are achieving the caloric deficit you need. It's a win-win.

But if this isn't happening for you, it may be time to make adjustments to your approach. To do this, you can use a technique I have been using in my clinic for years that I call the AIM process.

AIM FOR THE IDEAL COMBINATION OF EXERCISE AND DIET

AIM stands for:

- ✓ Assess
- ✓ Investigate
- ✓ Modify

By using this process, you will officially give up the mentality of a dieter and instead learn how to be a metabolic detective. Here is how it is done.

Assess

First review your SHMEC from the tracking worksheet in your *Metabolic Renewal Transformation Tracker*. SHMEC is in optimal balance when you score 20 on all five sensations for a total score of 100. The lower your score, the worse your metabolism is functioning.

After assessing SHMEC, you will want to check your fat loss. You will know if you are losing fat if the hourglass shape test that you take once a week is changing in desirable ways. You should be losing inches from the fatty places on your body. Over time you will also gain muscle in your thighs, chest, etc.

So, review your tracker and see if there is any change in those figures. It will be very clear to you whether or not you are losing fat.

Investigate

Now that you have your results for SHMEC and your fat-loss measurements, it is time to investigate your results. Did you get good results or poor results?

Remember, there are two things required for sustained and lasting fat loss: calorie reduction and hormonal balance. SHMEC tells you about hormonal balance and fat loss tells you about calories. Once you know where you stand, it is time to make modifications.

Modify

There are four possible outcomes to your SHMEC assessment and fat-loss tracking:

1. SHMEC is in check, and you are losing fat.
2. SHMEC is in check, but fat is not lost.
3. SHMEC is not in check, but you are losing fat.
4. SHMEC is not in check, and fat is not lost.

Depending on which of these outcomes applies to you, you will want to modify this program as follows.

#1: SHMEC IS IN CHECK, AND YOU ARE LOSING FAT

Congratulations! You have discovered the holy grail of body change. This means the program as outlined is working for you, and you don't need to make any changes.

However, there are two critical mistakes many make that I want you to avoid:

1. Do not try to speed things up by pushing your metabolism harder—you are more likely to push yourself right out of this balanced state.
2. Do not start looking for another way. We humans are funny; often when we find something that works, we promptly stop doing it. Your job now is practice, practice and more practice.

#2: SHMEC IS IN CHECK, BUT FAT IS NOT LOST

Some part of the program must be working for you, as you've gotten the hormonal balance side of the equation right—after all, your SHMEC is in check. But what if your SHMEC is in check, but your fat-loss results are either not coming or heading in the wrong direction? Surprisingly this is not as bad as you think. All you need to do is focus on the two biggest components of your nutrition that will increase calories and send your hormones out of balance: fat and starch.

Here is what I do with my patients when I encounter this scenario in my clinic:

1. Cut starchy foods back at each meal
2. Move all starch intake to one meal only (best at breakfast, dinner or post-workout)
3. Cut back on fat
4. Eat less frequently
5. Search for trigger foods
6. Start closely monitoring calories

Which of these steps work is highly individualized, so I encourage you to experiment. Try the first step for 7 to 14 days, and see if it works for you by tracking your SHMEC and fat loss. If it does, you've found the ticket. If not, move on to the next step, and so on until you find what works for you.

#3: SHMEC IS NOT IN CHECK, BUT YOU ARE LOSING FAT

You may think this is a desirable state, but it is the classic dieter's trap. It is alluring because you are getting some short-term results. But the fact that your SHMEC is out of check tells you that you are in metabolic compensation and will soon suffer the same fate as 95% of dieters—yo-yo weight regain.

Here's what to do to get your SHMEC in check and avoid the yo-yo diet trap:

1. Add more protein, fiber and water (such as lean protein and veggies)
2. Add in fat
3. Add in starch and subtract out fat
4. Add starch and fat
5. Add one or two snacks between meals

Again, you will need to experiment to see what works for you. Start with the first step and test it for 7-14 days. If it works, great. If not, move on to the second step, and so forth.

Don't be lazy about this. It's easy to think that if you are losing weight and your body shape is changing that all is good in the world. But until you get your SHMEC in check, there is no way you will be able to sustain your weight loss. I strongly encourage you to take these steps, and make sure you get your SHMEC in check. It's actually more important than fat loss.

#4: SHMEC IS NOT IN CHECK, AND FAT IS NOT LOST

Obviously, this is the worst of the scenarios and requires the most serious intervention. It can also happen for many different reasons. The first order of business is to get SHMEC in check. This is most important as obtaining hormonal balance is going to help you keep fat off long term. There's no point going to the work of burning fat if your hormones are out of balance.

So here are the steps you need to take to get SHMEC back in check.

1. Add more protein, fiber and water (such as lean protein and veggies)
2. Add in fat
3. Add in starch and subtract out fat
4. Add starch and fat
5. Add one or two snacks between meals

How much of each should you add? Again, that varies from person to person, but here are some guidelines:

- ✓ **Protein and Fiber**: Consider adding five more bites of each. That is about 4 ounces of protein or 20 grams and approximately eight ounces or one cup of vegetables.
- ✓ **Starch**: Consider adding three big bites of starch. That is about ½ cup or 15 grams.
- ✓ **Fat**: Consider adding one extra tablespoon or 10 grams.

Remember, stay flexible in your approach and be open to trial and error. There is no more important skill to have than this type of metabolic mastery. Once your SHMEC is in check, then you can start working on burning fat. Here are the steps to take:

1. Cut starchy foods back at each meal
2. Move all starch intake to one meal only (best at either breakfast, dinner or post-workout)
3. Cut back on fat
4. Eat less frequently
5. Search for trigger foods
6. Start closely monitoring calories

The bottom line is simply this: Most of you will be able to follow the diet plan for your cycle in Chapter 6, match that with the *Metabolic Renewal* exercise routines, and your fat-burning engines will shift into high gear. However, for a few of you it may take a little extra detective work to figure out the best eating plan for you. If your SHMEC is out of check, or you aren't losing fat within 14 days of starting this program, it's time to reassess and figure out what you need to change to find that fat-burning holy grail you are looking for.

It may take a little time and detective work, but I know you can make it happen.

WHAT YOU LEARNED IN THIS CHAPTER:

- ✓ We are all metabolically and hormonally different, and the idea that there is a one-size-fits all diet that works is simply wrong.
- ✓ That means you need to design a diet that works for you.
- ✓ That starts with the diet plans based on your hormone type in Chapter 6.
- ✓ Then, if you don't start seeing results in 7-14 days, use the AIM protocol to further tailor the program to your needs.

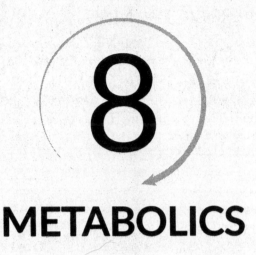

METABOLICS

Remember, when I refer to "metabolics" I am talking about things you do to intentionally influence the metabolism. This can include exercise, drugs and supplements. In this chapter we will focus on exercise specifically.

Here's the secret about exercise that almost no one realizes: Most people exercise too much and for too long. The key is intensity, efficiency and rest.

That's right, I said rest. Let me explain.

Any old type of exercise will burn calories. And pretty much any type of movement is healthy for you to do. But only certain forms of exercise force your body to change, adapt and turn on your fat-burning potential. To get this effect requires a unique form of metabolic intensity that not just any type of exercise can accomplish.

The magic is partly in the intensity. *Metabolic Renewal* is able to accomplish all of this because, unlike traditional cardio or slow-motion weight training, it breaches what exercise science calls the anaerobic threshold. This threshold is reached when exercise intensity becomes so high that the body is forced to mobilize resources in the moment and make metabolic alterations to meet the same or similar demands in the future.

This is why it blows traditional approaches away.

Traditional exercise, like cardio and weights, either don't get your body to reach this state at all or do not reach it long enough or frequently enough to make a difference. These old approaches may burn some calories—and muscle, too—but they don't always make much of a difference in the way you look.

Sure, if you run every day for miles or lift super intense weights, you may notice a few changes. If you are a runner, you will lose some fat, but you could lose muscle as well. Instead of getting the change you want, you can become skinny and flabby, and be a less efficient fat burner. If you lift weights, you may gain muscle but you probably won't burn much fat. You could wind up looking bulky. And again, you will only marginally change your ability to burn fat.

Neither of these scenarios are what people are after, yet they are so prevalent in the exercise world. To burn fat, sculpt muscle and change your fat-burning potential for good, there is a much better approach. Not just shorter and more intense, but one that is carefully structured and specifically tailored to your individual metabolism.

BETTER THAN ANAEROBIC TRAINING

Many studies have shown that shorter, more intense workouts burn fat more effectively. The following are just a few. There are literally dozens of studies out there that have shown similar results.

A study published in *Medicine and Science in Sports and Exercise* in 1996 showed that an anaerobic trained interval group burned significantly more fat than their aerobically trained counterparts.[16] Not only did the interval group burn greater amounts of fat during exercise, but they also exhibited increased fat burning effects that persisted for 24 hours after the exercise had stopped. The interval group was able to accomplish this with an exercise session that was a full 15 minutes shorter than the aerobic group.

Another study in the journal *Metabolism*[17] tracked two groups of people—one group doing aerobic training for a period of 20 weeks and another doing HIIT for 15 weeks. The researchers wanted to see how each program would impact body composition. The aerobic group burned 48 percent more calories than the interval group. However, the interval group enjoyed a **9-fold greater loss in subcutaneous fat**. At the conclusion of the study muscle biopsy analysis showed resting levels of 3-hydroxyacyl coenzyme A dehydrogenase (HADH), a marker of fatty acid oxidation, were significantly elevated in the interval group, but not the aerobic group.

A 2008 study in the *International Journal of Obesity* looked at intense intermittent exercise compared to steady state aerobics.[18] Forty-five healthy women between the ages of 18 and 30 were recruited for the study, divided into 3 groups, and studied for 15 weeks.

One group did HIIT, where they sprinted on a bike for 8 seconds followed by 12 seconds of rest. This was repeated for 20 minutes. Another group did moderately intense peddling that was sustained for 40 minutes. The final group did no exercise. At the end of the 15 weeks, the high- intensity interval group lost 2.5 pounds of fat while the steady-state aerobic group actually gained .6 pounds of fat. A measure of the fat-related hormones leptin and insulin were also positively affected in the HIIT group compared to the steady state group. This was accomplished with a workout that was half as long—20 minutes vs. 40 minutes.

BETTER THAN INTERVAL TRAINING

You may be familiar with some of these concepts through a training technique called interval training.[19] This technique has been growing in popularity because it is so much more effective than traditional exercise. It's more impactful because it makes use of some of the same physiological changes that *Metabolic Renewal* does. But it is not scalable to the individual. It works very well for those who are super fit and can do it, but most can't.

Metabolic Renewal puts interval training's positive effects on steroids by generating the cardiovascular component through fast-paced weight training and by teaching you to know when to rest and for how long. This takes *Metabolic Renewal* to an entirely different level.

And unlike interval exercise and aerobic fat-burning zone formulas, *Metabolic Renewal* is tailored to you. It adapts immediately to your fitness level and metabolic state. This means you will get more metabolic benefits from the workouts, the sessions will be safer, and you will recover much more quickly between sessions. The individual aspects of the sessions work so well that we have had elite athletes in the same sessions as seventy- and eighty-year-old grandparents.

How is this possible? The key is knowing when to rest and for how long. As you will hear me say over and over again in the exercise videos, "Rest is success in this program." I want you to rest. I *love it* when you rest. Here's why.

HUMANS CAN SELF-REGULATE EXERCISE, JUST LIKE OTHER ANIMALS

Did you ever have a pet hamster as a kid? If not, you've surely watched squirrels or other animals and seen this phenomenon: They run, they stop and rest, and then they run some more when they are ready. This is the essence of rest-based training, and it turns out that humans have this same built-in ability to regulate movement. We seem to know when to push hard and when to rest, just like other animals.

This was explained in a January 2011 study published in the journal *Psychophysiology*.[20] Researchers wanted to see how traditional interval training (where work-to-rest ratios were pre-set and standardized to be the same for everyone) compared to self-paced interval exercise (where work and rest intervals were self-defined by each participants).

Three different methods of gauging exercise intensity and recovery were used in this study:

1. **Heart rate recovery intervals:** Exercisers resumed exercise when the heart rate returned to 130 beats per minute.
2. **Defined rest intervals:** Exercisers resumed exercise after the rest period equaled the work period. A 1:1 work to rest interval ratio.
3. **Self-paced intervals:** Exercisers resumed exercise when they felt "ready."

The self-paced interval group performed slightly better, was shown to have worked just as hard as the traditional interval group, and finished the session slightly faster. The heart-rate recovery interval group had the lowest intensity levels.

Interval training is all about maximizing the work-to-rest ratio to maximize performance and intensity. Self-paced or rest-based interval training was able to accomplish a better outcome. Research has also shown rest-based or self-paced exercise is psychologically easier.[21,22,23,24,25]

The common notion that letting people self-select their exercise intensity and rest periods will result in less effective workouts is wrong. It actually makes the workouts more effective and more psychologically pleasing.

Traditional interval training is like someone grabbing your hand and sticking it on a hot stove, giving you little control of when it will be taken off. Naturally, you would resist this and there would be more of a chance of getting burned. But if you were free to quickly touch the stove and pull your hand off as fast as possible, or leave it on for as long as you felt comfortable, there would be no resistance necessary. Nor would you get burned.

We call rest-based training "interval training on steroids," because it gives you all the metabolic benefits of traditional interval training, but allows you to work even harder than you would otherwise since you are in complete control. Prioritizing rest over work is what allows this magical effect to happen. Harder work leads to more fat calories burned during exercise. And quality rest is required to produce quality work. It is win-win for the metabolism.

So how do you integrate this style of rest-based training into your life?

THE *METABOLIC RENEWAL* BASE EXERCISE PLAN

As with the nutrition program, we will start with a base exercise plan everyone can do, and then make modifications depending on where you are in your cycle and in your life.

The base plan is an ELEL approach and is simply this:

✓ Do the 15-minute routines on the videos that came with this program 3 times per week...

✓ And walk one to two hours on all or most days. This is about 5,000 to 10,000 steps per day.

Remember, walking is not exercise. Do it slowly and relax. It lowers cortisol and works synergistically with your exercise sessions. Most women do not need to do more than this. It simply isn't necessary, and overdoing it actually compromises your fat loss results in some cases.

CUSTOMIZING THE PROGRAM FOR YOUR FITNESS LEVEL

When you play the videos, there are a few things you will notice. First, you will see that there are three variations—one that is bodyweight only, one with bands and one with weights. Select the version that matches your fitness level.

If you have never done a workout like this before, you will probably want to start with the bodyweight-only versions. If you are a super-fit, go for the dumbbells. If you are somewhere in the middle, go for the bands. Test it out, and see what works for you.

If you try the bands or dumbbells don't get too caught up on them. Try to see this equipment as an extension of your body, and don't worry about perfect form so much.

The bands can be a bit tricky in some exercises and will require some experimenting. Watch the trainers to see if the position is correct. On many of the pressing movements you will want the bands behind the elbows. Another hint on the bands is that you may at times need to "choke up" on the band to get the correct tension. This is easily done by wrapping the band around your hand one or two times.

The dumbbells are far easier to manage. The major thing to remember with dumbbells is making sure that they are clear of your floor space when not in use during a workout. You don't want to inadvertently twist an ankle.

HOW TO CHOOSE THE RIGHT BANDS OR DUMBBELLS FOR YOU

Choose bands that allow you to do 5 to 10 repetitions with the weakest muscles that the bands will be used for. In this workout, those movements are going to be the side or rear shoulder raises. Choose a tension that allows you to complete at least 5 reps, but no more than 10 reps with these bands.

Keep in mind that if the bands you have chosen are too light, "choking up" on the bands by wrapping them around the hands one or two times works great.

For dumbbells, the same concept applies but the formula is slightly different. Start out by finding a 3-rep max for the weakest exercise you will encounter during metabolic prime. Again, that will be the side raise for most people.

A 3-rep max (3RM) is a weight you can do 3 times with good form, but not a fourth time. Find a 3RM on the dumbbell side raise exercise. Once you have found your weight, cut that weight in half. That is your weight for the workout.

For example, I can do 50 lbs. 3 times but not 4 on a dumbbell side raise. Fifty is my 3RM. Now I will divide that number by 2 to get the weight I will use for the workout, 25lbs.

The next thing you will notice is that there are burnout sessions for each workout. These 5-minute bonus routines are completely optional. They are designed to burn up a little extra fat. I encourage you to try them, but you don't have to do them. These are great for those of you fitness buffs who love to go for it.

Finally, you will see that even the super-ripped fitness instructors in these videos rest. If they need to rest, that means *you* are going to need to rest too. **Pushing to the point of rest is your goal in a rest-based workout.** I *do not* want you to pace. The mantra of *Metabolic Renewal* is this:

Push until you can't, then rest until you can.

I can't overstate the importance of this component of the program. Rest is the key to success. If you force yourself to go on or you start pacing yourself, you will not get the results you desire. These workouts are designed to *force* your body to rest. You should *never* feel guilty about taking too much rest. Sufficient recovery is the key to sufficient intensity.

For those of you who are just starting with this style of training, that may mean you are exercising for only a few minutes of the entire 15-minute workout. The remainder may be rest. Others who are more advanced may only rest for 2-3 minutes during the entire time. The amount you need to rest will naturally decrease as your overall fitness level and ability to recover increases.

> The key point is that the whole workout is only 15 minutes, INCLUDING rest, and you should rest as much as you need to. Do not pause the video to rest, keep it going and just pick back up when you are ready. The 15 minutes is truly 15 minutes of elapsed time, which includes both your exercise and your rest time.

This confuses people initially as they are used to pausing the workout video to rest and recover. That's one area where this workout is very different as the rest is a critical part of the overall workout. This is of critical importance, since the more you like the workout, the more consistent you can be. When you realize you have permission to rest, you will voluntarily work harder without even being consciously aware you are doing so.

That's really all there is to it. Watch the videos. Follow along. Push hard. Rest hard. Try to do the burnouts. Cool down with a walk after the workout is over. However, if you want to dial this in a little further and take your results to another level, you can modify the program to fit with your cycle and where you are in your life as follows.

EXERCISE MODIFICATIONS FOR MENSTRUATING WOMEN

If you are a younger woman and you menstruate normally, start with the exercise videos as noted above. However, in the follicular phase (the first two weeks) of your cycle you can take an EMEM approach—adding more workouts to your plan. Here's why:

During the follicular phase estrogen is rising and more dominant. Estrogen makes the body more stress-resistant. It also will allow you to get a little more fat burning and muscle building out of your workouts, the same way testosterone works for men.

Combine this with the HGH-stimulating effects of the Renewal workouts, and you have a perfect hormonal mixture for optimizing fat loss and muscle shaping. You don't have to do more during this phase of your cycle to see great results, but some women may want to. If you want to try this cycling approach, here is what you do.

1. Do the *Metabolic Renewal* workouts three times a week as usual.
2. Add up to three additional workouts per week.

It's as simple as that. Here are some options for the additional workouts:

✓ **Extra *Metabolic Renewal* workouts.** You can repeat the *Metabolic Renewal* workouts (do them up to 6 times per week instead of 3 times per week).

✓ **Cardio-centered workouts (intervals or traditional cardio).** Take a single cardio activity (running, rowing, biking, jumping rope, calisthenics or any other cardio-centered activity) and add a few of these workouts in to the regimen if you wish to and find them enjoyable.

✓ **Your personal favorite.** Do you love yoga or Pilates? CrossFit? Are you a runner? If you already have an activity you love, now is the time to add it in and really push it.

✓ **Do the burnouts or add weights.** This is another way to increase the intensity during your follicular phase. Try adding in the burnouts or do the routines with weights if you don't already.

✓ **Any combination of these.** Maybe you want to add one cardio workout, one yoga workout and one additional *Metabolic Renewal* workout. That's totally fine as well. The key is finding a combination of workouts that you'll enjoy and look forward to.

The point of all of this is to leverage the fat-burning potential during the follicular phase of your cycle in a way you enjoy and makes sense for you. That part is very important. Do what you love. Don't make yourself run if you hate it. Find something you enjoy and add that to your plan.

Now, there are a few additional tips I have for you based on your hormone type. Let's check them out.

Normal Menstrual Cycle—Estrogen and Progesterone Balanced

Your metabolism is balanced and cyclical, and as a result you can better tolerate exercise in general. What may work best for you is splitting time between EMEM for the first two weeks of your cycle and ELEL for last two weeks. You may want to consider adding three traditional weight-training workouts during your EMEM times. This will provide the most substantial and pronounced results in terms of tone and tightness.

Normal Menstrual Cycle—Estrogen Dominant

Because estrogen has effects similar to testosterone, allowing you to be less impacted by stress, you may want to consider adding additional cardio workouts during your EMEM phase (the first two weeks of your cycle). This can amplify some of the fat loss you will achieve and your more estrogen dominant state may allow you to handle it better.

Also, because cardio workouts typically induce more sweating than weightlifting workouts, and sweating is a prime mechanism by which the body gets rid of estrogen-mimicking pollutants, try to work up a good sweat. This means upping the temperature in your workout area and avoiding fans. A good sweat is a great way to detox from exogenous estrogens.

Normal Menstrual Cycle—Progesterone Deficient

Because estrogen and progesterone work together to keep cortisol levels down and progesterone is the first to fall during times of stress, including exercise stress, you may want to keep your extra workouts short.

Adding three very short high-intensity interval training sessions during your EMEM times (the first two weeks of your cycle) can be a great approach for you. These workouts are intense, yes, but they are also short and minimize stress. This is a great approach for this hormone.

Normal Menstrual Cycle—Estrogen and Progesterone Deficient

Stress is your major nemesis and you want to be extra careful to help your body rest and recover. It is a great idea for you to add relaxing and restorative exercise sessions like yoga, Pilates, or Tai Chi during your EMEM (the first two weeks of your cycle). These will still give you a good workout, but also allow you to work on some of the relaxing aspects of things, by breathing, stretching and training your ability to relax and be present.

EXERCISE MODIFICATIONS FOR PERIMENOPAUSE, MENOPAUSE AND POST-MENOPAUSE

I have two recommendations for women in this phase of life when it comes to exercise.

First, walking is more important than your workouts. Actually, this is probably true for everyone, but it's especially important for menopausal women. Remember, your body is more stress reactive at this time of life. Walking is one of the only forms of physical exercise you can do that is actually a stress reducer.

So please don't underestimate this part of the program. I'd rather see you follow the nutrition plan and walk one to two hours a day on all or most days than train intensely and stress yourself out even further.

Which leads to my second recommendation: If you need to, you can dial the base plan back a little by only working out twice per week. For most women, this won't be necessary. But if you find your SHMEC remains out of balance, you have worked through the AIM protocol in Chapter 7, and you feel stressed out, this may be a sign that you are overdoing it on exercise.

If your metabolism can handle it and SHMEC remains in check, do the *Metabolic Renewal* workouts three times per week. If you find SHMEC goes out of check, try scaling back to only two *Metabolic Renewal* workouts per week and see how that goes.

And keep the following in mind when it comes to your specific hormone type:

Perimenopause—Estrogen Fluctuating, Progesterone Deficient

Because there are times when your estrogen is up and then down and because your body finds itself in a new metabolic reality of low progesterone, this is one of the most stressful times of a woman's life. You will want to pay extra attention to any kind of activity or exercise that helps to lower stress hormones.

I suggest yoga, Pilates or new modalities like MovNat or Animal Flow on days off from the renewal workouts. These should not get you out of breath and should feel relaxed and easy. Not all yoga classes are created equal, so make sure you find the ones that feel like nap time versus yoga time.

Menopause—Estrogen and Progesterone Deficient

At this point you are likely beginning to see a shift of fat storage around the middle despite no or little change in what you are eating. It is important that you don't try to over-exercise to compensate for this. That will just stress you out further and ironically make matters worse.

One great approach you can use is to simply make sure you take a nice long walk for 30 to 60 minutes after your workouts. By timing this walk right after a workout you will be able to lower cortisol and further burn fat released during the workout.

Post-Menopause—Estrogen and Progesterone Deficient

You are dealing with a unique condition where estrogen and progesterone are low and testosterone, while it may be lower as well, is still higher relative to what it was previously. This can lead to a metabolic state that may cause reduced muscle mass and bone mineral density.

As a result of this, you will want to pay extra attention to using weights heavy enough to challenge your system. There are several ways you can do this. You can increase the weights you use during your workouts. You can consider adding one or two separate weight training only workouts and/or do loaded walks by putting 20 to 40 pounds in a backpack and walking for 60 minutes 2 to 4 times per week.

All of this will coax your body into developing more lean tissue, adding fat loss, and decreasing the risk of bone loss, falling and fractures.

EXERCISE MODIFICATIONS FOR SPECIAL CASES

The great thing about this program is that it can work for all kinds of special cases as well: pregnancy, post-pregnancy and various kinds of metabolic challenges. So let's look at each of these situations.

THE PREGNANT WOMAN

The idea that a healthy pregnant woman should be resting in bed is ridiculous. Do you think our pregnant ancestors laid down for nine to ten months? Not on your life.

Pregnancy is not the time to start exercising like crazy if you have not been, but it is also not the time to stop if you have been. With the right modifications (more on this below), many of the routines in this program can be done by pregnant women. However, if this is your first time considering rest-based interval training, I would wait until after baby is born to start following the videos in earnest.

One great strategy to use if you are not used to exercise is to do the walking along with a light, non-weighted version of the workouts (meaning bodyweight only). In this approach, you follow along with the workouts without weights and move through the exercises slowly, almost like you would see someone move if they were doing tai chi. This slow movement will provide benefit to you and the baby with little risk. Obviously, if you are an exerciser this workout is perfect to do after speaking with your doctor.

A few guidelines to keep in mind: During the first trimester minimize intense jumping exercises. Just take them out and do a non-jumping version. For example, squat jumps just turn into squats. During the third trimester avoid any exercise that has you laying on your stomach or crunching on the abdomen. This is pretty obvious at this point in the pregnancy, but it bears mentioning. If you are breastfeeding, you can enjoy the workouts just as is. You may want to wear a little more breast support if you experience tenderness in that area.

Whatever you choose, I strongly encourage you to speak with your physician about your particular situation.

THE METABOLICALLY CHALLENGED WOMAN

Metabolic Renewal is specifically designed to awaken the sleeping metabolism. I can't think of a better program for women with metabolic challenges like hypothyroidism, PCOS and others. However, there are a few things to keep in mind if you are metabolically challenged. Exercise can be your greatest ally in getting your metabolism back, but it also can be too much too soon.

One way you can tailor this program to fit your needs is to use your heart rate recovery as a guide. After an intense bout of movement the heart rate will spike. When you take your rest it will fall. The degree to which it quickly spikes and falls is a window into the balance of your sympathetic and parasympathetic nervous systems.

Optimally, your heart rate should fall at least 20 beats in 1 minute after intense exertion. If this doesn't happen, it usually is an indication that your metabolism is overtaxed and has had enough for the day.

Often in those with chronic fatigue, fibromyalgia or other issues, this will start out being the case, and then at some point in the workout stop being the case. Stopping your workout at the point where your heart rate is no longer dropping quickly can be an extra guide for those who know exercise often wipes them out. This keeps you in the safe zone.

Now you know how to modify the base plan to your personal needs. However, there are a few other things I want to explain before we move on.

THE IMPORTANCE OF FORM

When it comes to performing the exercises in *Metabolic Renewal*, there are a few things you should be aware of. We are all uniquely different and this applies to our level of fitness and physical abilities. Some of us have current or past injuries making it difficult to perform certain exercises. Some of us have athletic backgrounds and a refined level of coordination, and some of us don't.

One of the biggest mistakes people make with exercise is overly focusing on these considerations. Despite what you have been told, there is no perfect way to do each exercise. There are generalizations, and you should try to duplicate the form exhibited by the trainers in the videos as much as you are able to. However, you should also allow your body some leeway in terms of how it moves.

If you need to adjust the exercises in any way, do not be afraid to do that. I'll tell you more about how to do that in a moment, but first I want to share a realization I've had about exercise form over the years.

Moving More Almost Always Leads to Moving Better

Your body improves at exercise when you exercise. Coordination and balance come from actually exercising. You don't become proficient at squats from being hypervigilant over the way you are squatting. The best way to become proficient at squats is to simply do more squats, and let your body learn the rhythm of the movement.

There was an old story I heard where a pottery instructor told her students to make the perfect pot. Half of the class was instructed on how to make the pot and told to focus making the best pot. The other half of the class was told to make as many pots as possible. After a period of time the class presented their pots to be judged. Guess who won? The group that was instructed to just make lots of pots had succeeded in not only making more pots, but also in making better pots.

In other words, practice makes perfect. The more opportunity you have to move, the better you will be able to move. This is almost always the case with exercise. So give yourself permission to move more, even if the exercise is not completely perfect just yet. Your body will "get it" in time, and it will happen faster than stressing over every little angle of movement.

With this in mind we can now talk about how to adapt this program to your specific needs.

Regressions and Progressions

In the field of exercise we have ways to make exercises easier. We call these regressions. We also have ways of making exercises harder. These are called progressions.

Let's use a push-up as an example for regression. You can do a push-up on your toes. You can regress the push-up down a level by doing it from your knees. You can go down another level by doing the push-up off a wall. You can even regress one more level still by rolling over on your back and doing a chest press with light dumbbells.

On the other end of the spectrum we have progressions. Let's use the squat as an example. You can do a regular body weight squat. You can progress that by holding bands and doing a band-weighted squat.

The exercise can be progressed again by using dumbbells. It can be progressed further by doing a one-legged squat or adding a heavy barbell.

You should feel absolutely free to regress or progress an exercise to a level that fits you. In this program you will see that I have already added a level of regression and progression that you can choose. The bodyweight exercises are easiest. The bands progress it one level and dumbbells add another level of progression. The trick is to use your judgment as to which degree of resistance you will use and which exercise regression or progression best suits you.

I obviously can't outline every possible option for every possible person, nor would I want to. You know your body better than I do. Tune into it and listen to what it's telling you. Do what works for you. However, if you need more assistance on learning specifically how to progress or regress an exercise to fit your needs, we have a special bonus for you.

In the videos you received, you will find a dedicated segment where I show you how to progress and regress the major movements in the program. Check that out, listen to your body, and adjust these exercises to fit your needs.

WHAT IF YOU ARE OVERWEIGHT OR HAVE INJURIES?

One question I get all the time is, "What do I do if I have an injury?" or "What if I am overweight?" The answer to these questions is very simple, although not always something people like to hear.

If you have bad knees, then work out using your arms and skip the leg exercises. If you have injured shoulders, then go lighter on the arm stuff (or avoid it altogether) and just focus on the legs. Can't use your right arm? Then use your left. Can't use the left? Use the right. In other words, move the body parts you are able to use. It may surprise you to know that research suggests that moving the non-injured limb actually does have some benefit in strengthening the limb you can't move. This has to do with "nervous system crossover."

If you are overweight and have difficulty moving up and down off the floor, I encourage you to do it anyway. One of the most demanding, useful and metabolically stimulating activities an overweight person can engage in is getting up and down off the floor. In some ways, this is more beneficial than almost any other exercise.

You may notice that I have purposely programmed things in a way that requires up and down movements. They are so effective, and that is why I like to take advantage of them. So don't feel defeated if you are slow to get up and down—instead, pat yourself on the back and realize that you are getting a more effective workout than you would otherwise.

METABOLIC CHAINS

One of the things you will notice about *Metabolic Renewal* is the specific design of the exercises and other workout elements. The workout makes judicious use of several techniques all designed to generate the Bs and Hs—breathless, burning, heavy and heat.

For women, two of these four are more important than the others: breathless and burning. When a workout generates these two sensations simultaneously it is an indication of adrenaline and HGH release. These hormones work synergistically with estrogen and progesterone to create the lean beautiful hourglass shape the female form is known for.

One of the cornerstone techniques is called "metabolic chains." These are exercises that string separate movements into one single activity. You can think of the separate exercises as one link in the chain. Then one or more of the links is "compacted" by adding reps each time. This is a devastatingly effective way to increase the density of a workout.

The *Metabolic Renewal* workouts are dense because they stuff a crazy volume of exercise into such a short period of time. This is one of the key reasons they have such a beneficial metabolic effect. Achieving this density would be nearly impossible to do without the metabolic chain system.

The other thing that is great about metabolic chains is that you have to keep your own rep count. You might think that is because I am lazy and don't want to count for you, but in reality, it is a key part of keeping you focused on extrinsic factors, rather than intrinsic feelings. This is a sleight-of-hand tactic I use to get you to push a little harder without even realizing.

There are a few subsets of the metabolic chains as well. You will also be using "rep chains" and "squeeze chains."

REPS CHAINS

Rep chains alter a single exercise's range of motion in a series. On the first round, you do one of each movement, on the second round you do two of each movement, on the third round you do three of each movement, and, finally, on the fourth round you do four of each movement. Then you reset back to one and work your way up to four again. This is repeated again and again as many times as possible in the allotted time.

An example of rep chains that you will encounter in the workout is the push-up rep chain. In this case, each rep variation is a link in the chain and each can be added to or "compacted" each time through the sequence. You also alter the range of motion so that you can keep more tension on the muscles and achieve more vascular occlusion (a concept I discuss below).

For example, the push-up rep chain consists of three different movements:

1. Bottom to ¼ of the way up (a "pulsing rep")
2. Bottom to ½ of the way up (a "half rep")
3. Bottom to the top (a "full rep")

To complete the push-rep chain, do as follows:

✓ **Round 1** = 1 pulsing rep, 1 half rep, 1 full rep
✓ **Round 2** = 2 pulsing rep, 2 half rep, 2 full rep
✓ **Round 3** = 3 pulsing rep, 3 half rep, 3 full rep
✓ **Round 4** = 4 pulsing rep, 4 half rep, 4 full rep

Then you start back at round 1, and on it goes until the allotted time expires. As always in rest-based training, you rest whenever you need to and then begin again right where you left off. These rep chains sequences are powerful metabolic stimulators and unique in the exercise world.

SQUEEZE CHAINS

Squeeze chains use seconds as links in the chain instead of reps. The movement stays exactly the same, you just hold it for varying lengths of time. An example of the squeeze chains you will see in this program is the shoulder front-raise squeeze chain. This exercise is deceptively simple, but done right, you'll be burning, sweating and breathing heavy in no time.

To do this exercise, you simply raise your arms out in front of your body, bringing them up to shoulder height. At this point, you squeeze your fists, chest, shoulders upper arms and forearms as tight as you can. At the top of the first rep you hold the squeeze for one second. On the second rep you hold for a count of two seconds. The third round is a three-second hold and squeeze. Finally, the fourth round is held for four seconds. You then go back to a one-second hold before working your way up the squeeze chain again.

And on it goes until the time for that movement expires. Just as with rep chains, you should always keep in mind that this is rest-based training, so you should rest when you need it, then start again when you are ready, right where you left off.

The *Metabolic Renewal* chains use a four count. That means they are compacted only up to four before starting over again. Rep and squeeze chains help generate more burning and make use of vascular occlusion.

VASCULAR OCCLUSION

Another thing you will notice about the *Metabolic Renewal* workout that is different from other types of exercise is the use of squeezing, tension reps, holding reps and other techniques designed to produce burning. These workout techniques make use of how the body circulates blood. Blood moves through your arteries due to the pressure created by the pumping heart, and because arteries contain small muscles that can push and squeeze the blood along.

Once the blood gets into your capillaries and drops off its nutrients and oxygen to your working muscles, it enters your veins to return to the heart. But veins don't get the benefit of the beating heart, and they are not lined with muscles. Veins rely on your skeletal muscle. When your muscle contracts and relaxes, this acts like a pump to move blood along. Veins also contain valves so the blood can't move backwards.

When you squeeze down on a muscle by contracting and holding it, or do not allow it to completely relax, you are holding the blood in place for a longer period of time and slowing its return to the heart. You may think this is a bad thing, but the muscles are constantly releasing signaling molecules that are carried away by the blood to distant areas.

You can think of these molecules as metabolic smoke signals. These compounds speak to your muscle, fat, brain and liver cells, and send signals for optimizing performance, recovery, repair and adaptation. The longer they are hanging around your muscles, the more time they have to stimulate beneficial fat-burning and muscle-sculpting events in those muscles.

You know you are creating the effect when your muscles burn and feel swollen and heavy (called the muscle pump). When scientists study these techniques in the laboratory, they slow blood flow by applying tourniquets, like that little rubber strip that the nurse wraps around your arm when drawing blood.[26]

In the *Metabolic Renewal* workouts, we use squeezing, holding and tension reps to duplicate this effect. Dumbbells and bands take vascular occlusion to another level, which is why they are included for the more advanced practitioners. When you do this workout you will immediately feel something different compared to any other workout you have ever done. That is the vascular occlusion effect and it is best achieved when you focus hard on the squeezing I will ask you to do during some of your workouts.

That's all you need to know to get started with the exercise program in *Metabolic Renewal*. Go check out the videos and get after it!

WHAT YOU LEARNED IN THIS CHAPTER:

✓ The base exercise plan is simply to follow the videos. This means you will be doing rest-based interval training 3 times a week for 15 minutes and walking one to two hours on all or most days.

✓ If you are a normally menstruating woman, you can add additional exercise in the follicular phase of your cycle.

✓ Menopausal women may need to dial the program back a little, and only do it 2 times per week. Follow your SHMEC. It will tell you what to do. And make sure you get your walking in.

✓ Pregnant women can do the program as is, if they are already fit. If you are not an exerciser already, slow the program down or wait until post-pregnancy.

✓ If you are metabolically challenged, use your heart rate recovery as a guide to how much you should exercise.

MINDSET

O ne of the most prevalent questions I get asked goes something like this, "Dr. Jade, I have done everything right and I am still not losing weight. Why?" The answer is simple to me, but complex for everyone else. It is simple to me, because I have had the benefit of working with thousands of people over several decades. This gives me a unique perspective.

These people who say they have been "doing everything right" are typically focused on meals (what and how they are eating) and metabolics (exercise). What they miss is movement and mindset. We will discuss movement in Chapter 10. Here I want to talk about the critical importance of mindset.

The human body is one big stress barometer. Everything your metabolism does is designed to do one major thing—measure and react to stress. It is the metabolism's prime directive. Your mindset around stress is so important and almost no one pays any attention to it.

How many people do you know who say to themselves, "I am having trouble losing weight, I should take a nap or a hot bath or go have some relaxing sex?" Usually they are doing the exact opposite, aren't they? "I need to take this supplement, drink this magic elixir, exercise twice daily doing the new tangerine theory interval workout and eat nothing but organic kale and wild line-caught salmon."

Stress is the thing. Mindset around a lifestyle of rest, recovery and relaxation is the cure. Let's talk about stress and why it can kill your results.

HOW STRESS CAN KILL YOUR RESULTS

How many calories does stress have? I agree that this is a ridiculous question, but ask almost any health and fitness expert if stress can make a person fat and you will hear a resounding "yes." But if we agree that stress has no calories, and we also believe that fat gain is about nothing but calories, then how in the world does stress stimulate fat gain?

The truth is that the calorie model is not the whole story on fat loss. Stress and other lifestyle factors work through complicated hormonal and metabolic mechanisms that alter not only the amount of calories we eat, but also where on the body we store them and most importantly which type we burn—sugar, fat or muscle.

I realize not everyone likes to delve into the deep biochemistry that is required to truly understand how stress causes fat gain, so I will do my best to make this as simple as I can.

A Historical Frame of Reference

Before I can even begin to talk about stress, it is important to understand what it is and how humans have adapted to deal. Humans have evolved on this planet for millions of years. We have had to deal with predators, food shortages, ice ages, natural disasters, rugged terrain, an uncertain future and countless other "stressful" things.

If you think you have it tough today, imagine walking down the street and having a pack of hungry wolves jump out from behind a dumpster and decide you are dinner. Or walking into a grocery store where the cashier hands you a spear and points you towards the wild boar living in aisle 4. This may seem laughable right now, but understanding the physiological reaction of that kind of stress is exactly what is needed to decipher the impact stress has on fat gain.

The bottom line is that humans are designed for acute stress like running away from a hungry predator, fighting off an intruder, or catching dinner. That is because during the millions of years we have been on the planet, we encountered these stressors all the time.

Your physiology is hard-wired to the realities of your historic ancestors. Whether you are being chased by a pack of wolves, fighting a wild boar, under a severe deadline at work, facing financial uncertainty, or stuck in traffic, your response to stress is exactly the same as far as your physiology is concerned.

The Brain-Adrenal Axis

The stress response is regulated by a closely orchestrated communication between the hypothalamus, the pituitary gland and your adrenal glands. Is this starting to sound familiar? There is that HPA again. You can begin to see how it controls so many functions in the body.

You can think of the brain as an army's central command center. When it gets a warning that there is an incoming threat, it sends an immediate signal to the adrenal glands. In a fraction of a second, the adrenal glands flood the body with hormonal signals like adrenaline, noradrenaline, and cortisol, whose job is to give the body the energy required to stay and fight or run like hell.

You know what this feels like. If you have ever been in or near a car accident, you probably felt an intense surge of energy travel through your body that allowed you to slam on the brakes or swerve out of the way. That was your HPA axis in action. This is where things can go wrong.

In the modern day there is nothing to run from and there is no giant Twinkie monster you have to kill to get lunch. So instead of moving in response to stress, you just sit there with large amounts of adrenal hormones surging through your body. This is not a good thing.

The major action of adrenal hormones is to raise the amount of sugar and fat in the blood to supply the body with energy. The whole body mobilizes all at once to supply the body with everything it needs to survive. The liver is instructed to kick out stored sugar as well as make some extra. Muscle and fat aid the creation of new sugar through the release of amino acids from muscle and glycerol from triglyceride (fat) respectively.

In other words, stress burns fat, sugar and muscle under normal circumstances. But when it becomes recurrent and chronic, fat is usually spared while muscle is taken. Historically, when your body became stressed out, you were able to run your way to safety or fight your way out of danger. The process of intense movement to run away or fight is just what the body needs, because that triggers the release of other hormones like testosterone and human growth hormone (HGH).

Those hormones act to repair damaged tissue and partition energy usage towards fat metabolism while at the same time sparing and even building muscle. The repair mechanisms of these two hormones rebuild the body leaner, faster and stronger, improving the chances that the next stressful encounter will result in another success.

All of this together feeds back on the brain and the adrenals allowing them to stop the alarms and go back to a rest and recovery physiology.

Chronic Stress

The problem starts when stress, whether real or perceived, becomes constant and continuous, is not followed by intense activity, is not controlled through relaxing walking, or never ends. Chronic stress is different, because the stressors continually force the body to work harder and harder to compensate for the physiological disruptions.

One of the first and most important things to change is the relative amounts of cortisol in your blood. Relative is an important term, because it means how much cortisol you have in relation to other hormones.

The most important thing to remember here is that cortisol (one of your major stress hormones) exerts actions on the body that are beyond your awareness. High amounts of continuous cortisol secretion induce serious changes in our physiology. Two important changes occur in relation to hunger and cravings. Excess cortisol impacts hunger and increases the urge for sweets and fatty foods. A sure sign that you have high-stress levels is a lack of appetite in the morning.

Two studies, one in *Endocrinology*[27] and another other in *Psychoneuroendocrinology*,[28] show how cortisol can decrease hunger in the short term and increase binge eating with a desire for highly palatable foods later. In other words, cortisol makes you eat less often, but makes you overeat the wrong foods when you get the chance.

This makes complete sense when you think about stress from a historic perspective. If walking out of your house could result in you getting swept away by a giant pterodactyl, you would likely make fewer trips to the grocery store and seek out the most energy-dense foods to sustain you for longer. In other words, you would eat less frequently and avoid the danger lurking outside as much as possible.

A comprehensive review by Dr. Pecoraro of UCLA San Francisco was published in 2006 in the journal *Progress in Neurobiology*. In that paper, he cites research that shows that this is exactly the case.[29]

This review shows that through several overlapping mechanisms, chronic stress caused animals to decrease the number of times they ate, opting for a few big meals over lots of smaller ones. Stress also forces a preferential desire for sugar and fat over regular mixed composition meals.

The study shows that this happens at the level of the brain, because glucocorticoids, like cortisol, affect brain chemicals, specifically dopamine and opioids. These can lead towards depression or anxiety, lack of motivation, lack of spontaneous movement and a desire for high- calorie foods. Sounds a lot like what we call "emotional eating," right?

The bottom line here is that stress, when chronic and persistent, affects brain chemistry in a way that changes behavior. These behaviors are directly correlated to obesity and appear to be coming from more unconscious centers of the brain.

Stress and Women

Stress is definitely a menace when it comes to metabolism, and it is even more an issue for women. You have to remember that your metabolism is a stress barometer, and, as a woman, one of the major things it is measuring is the safety of diverting resources to reproduction.

If the metabolism deems things are "too stressful," it begins to down-regulate the female hormones. Typically progesterone drops first, which removes some of a woman's ability to cope with stress and begins to make estrogen less effective as well (progesterone primes estrogen receptors and vice versa.)

Next estrogen falls, leaving the female metabolism exposed to the full onslaught of cortisol and chronic stress as described above. This is one of the reasons I say that taking diet and exercise to the extreme is a huge contributing factor in lack of results in body change, and may be the major cause of fat gain or the inability to lose fat.

What is a woman to do? Listen to your body, and consider where you are in your life and your hormone type.

MINDSET MODIFICATIONS FOR MENSTRUATING WOMAN

The body handles stress in unique ways, and one of the ways it can impact some people is to make the metabolic seesaw shift in unexpected ways. This causes the command and control center of your metabolism—your hypothalamus – to send signals to the thyroid, adrenal glands and ovaries. This can compromise your hormones even further, and you can end up in a downward spiral of metabolic dysfunction.

If you are a younger woman with a normal cycle, your estrogen and progesterone levels are exquisitely attuned to this, and that can be a problem. We live in an environment that is stress-heavy, and most of us typically prioritize doing more and going harder over resting appropriately and working smarter.

I like to think of the ovarian system as a woman's most sensitive stress barometer. As stress levels rise, ovarian function becomes compromised. This results in falling progesterone, fluctuating estrogen, and then complete ovarian fatigue.

What you need to do is adjust your 4Ms so that you are reducing stress exposure, combatting stress excess (through relaxing and restorative behaviors) and not overdoing diet and exercise, which you may be prone to do.

There are many things you can do to reduce stress: meditation, massage, naps, sleep, hot baths, sauna, tai chi, relaxing stretching and more. (You'll learn more in this chapter.) However, there are some specific activities that can benefit your stress levels depending on your hormone type.

Normal Menstrual Cycle—Estrogen and Progesterone Balanced

In your case stress is not much of an issue in the first half of the month, but begins to really make an impact in the weeks leading up to menses. To help balance that we want to do things to decrease stress, especially in the premenstrual period.

There are two things that might be especially useful for you, and they are walking in nature and warm Epsom salt baths. Research has shown that relaxed, slow-paced walking is able to lower stress and that doing this in green areas is even better.[30] The Japanese even have a name for this. They call it *shirin-yoku* or "forest bathing."

When you add Epsom salt to your bath it takes an already wonderfully relaxing activity and puts its stress-reducing effects on overdrive. Epsom salt is magnesium sulfate and magnesium is very relaxing to the nervous system.

Both of these things dramatically counter stress and keep the hunger and cravings at bay.

Here is what I want you to do: In the two weeks leading up to menses, I want you to take either a 30 to 90 minute walk, preferably in a green setting, or take a bath. Do this every day and you will be priming your metabolism to respond in a way you never imagined.

Normal Menstrual Cycle—Estrogen Dominant

There are many ways you can become estrogen dominant. Regardless of how it happens, decreasing stress will help you rebalance your estrogen levels.

There is one thing that might be especially useful for you, and that is hot baths and/or sauna therapy. These therapies get you sweating, which is one of the main ways you get rid of some of the persistent organic pollutants that can have estrogen-like effects in the body.

Here is what I want you to do: Begin taking a hot bath or sauna, hot enough to get you sweating but cool enough to remain relaxing and allow you to sweat lightly for 20 to 60 minutes. Do this at least three times per week and preferably five or six times per week.

Normal Menstrual Cycle—Progesterone Deficient

In your case, this command-and-control signal may be getting jumbled a bit because progesterone levels are required to keep this entire system prime and sensitized. If progesterone levels fall, this system can become less dependable and more prone to issues.

To help balance that we want to do things to decrease stress or lessen its effects. This is the best way to maintain adequate progesterone levels.

However, there is one thing that might be especially useful for you, and that is learning to use your breath to adjust your physiology as needed. You can calm your mind by focusing on your breathing. This can produce a relaxation response in your brain and body that will wipe the stress away.

The technique I want you to do involves taking ten deep breath and four steps:

- ✓ Count eight seconds on the inhale
- ✓ Hold your breath for two seconds
- ✓ Exhale for four seconds
- ✓ After completing these ten breaths, close your eyes, take a big deep breath in, and hold it for as long as you comfortably can

Use this time to reset your senses and still your mind. Listen to your heartbeat or watch the color changes dance around in the back of your eyelids. Repeat this up to three times per day, including before bed to help you sleep.

Normal Menstrual Cycle—Estrogen and Progesterone Deficient

In your case the command-and-control signal has either lost its ability to communicate to the ovaries, or the ovaries have lost their ability to respond. It is almost always a combination of both, but most issues start in the brain and end in the ovaries.

That is why we want to do things to decrease stress and reduce its effects on the brain first. This is the best way to reboot the ovarian system and get estrogen and progesterone back in line.

Getting your body in restorative relaxation mode is going to be the key. Think of this as a reboot to your metabolic hard drive. The best way to do that is to sleep. There is only one problem, of all the hormonal types you may have the most difficult time getting to sleep at night. To combat this, you can use two other reboot techniques alongside sleep—naps and meditation.

Research shows that even a 10 to 30 minute nap can undo many of the hormonal problems caused by sleep loss.[31] Meditation has also been shown to restore function in the body and brain similar to how a nap does. By focusing on your breath, I mean counting the breaths. In, then out, that's one. Continue focusing on and counting your breath until you reach a count of 10, then start back over at one.

If your mind wanders and you forget your count, just go back to one. The counting allows you to catch your mind when it drifts. By the way, mental drift is normal in meditation, and with practice you can focus for much longer.

I want you to prioritize sleep by taking three steps:

- ✓ First, go to bed one hour earlier and rise one hour later to start. Shoot for 9 hours of sleep every night.
- ✓ Second, I want you to take a brief 10 to 20 minute nap between the hours of noon and 4:00 pm five days a week.
- ✓ Finally, I want you to meditate for 5 minutes by focusing on your breath at least 3 times per week.

MINDSET MODIFICATIONS FOR PERIMENOPAUSE, MENOPAUSE AND POST-MENOPAUSE

Due to fluctuating estrogen and falling progesterone during this time of life, your entire system is forever losing its cyclical rhythm. This means that you are now becoming more sensitive to fat storage from food and more reactive to fat storage from stress. It's a double whammy.

Learning how to cope with stress more effectively is essential. That being said, the modern Western lifestyle has a completely dysfunctional attitude toward stress. It is crucial that you do things to reduce your stress load. You can try meditation, massage, naps, sleep, hot baths, sauna, tai chi, relaxing stretching and a lot more.

However, I do have specific suggestions based on your hormone type.

Perimenopause—Estrogen Fluctuating, Progesterone Deficient

One thing that might be especially useful for you are social activities with friends while engaging in relaxing treatments like spa facials, pedicures and massages. Social support is critical during this time of life as it helps buffer against some of the unpredictable symptoms that come up.

Spending more time with friends going through the same thing is a great way to vent, connect and reduce stress. Try doing this while getting your nails done, getting a massage or doing anything you can do to treat yourself and relax. You'll get double the benefit. Plan at least two to four relaxing social outings with friends and/or family per week. Walking groups are great for this, as are creative groups like book clubs or other creative outlets.

In addition, I want you to engage in spa treatments as much as possible—at least three times per week. I realize this can become an issue in terms of time and finances, and I don't want you to stress.

If finances are an issue, look for lower-cost alternative such as self-massage and stretching classes (like restorative yoga).

Menopause—Estrogen and Progesterone Deficient

As estrogen and progesterone levels drop, your already exquisitely attuned stress barometer gets even more sensitive, because you become more reactive to the stress hormone cortisol. Reducing stress is the best way to deal with this new reality of reduced estrogen and progesterone. But our society doesn't make that easy.

Probably the most important thing a woman in your time of life can do to get her body in restorative relaxation mode is to get enough sleep. Sleep is like a reboot to your metabolic hard drive. There is only one problem: you may have a great difficulty falling asleep at night due to your changing hormones. To combat this you can use two other reboot techniques alongside sleep—naps and meditation.

Research shows that even a 10 to 30 minute nap can undo many of the hormonal problems caused by sleep loss.[32] Meditation has also been shown to restore function in the body and brain similar to a nap.

I want you to prioritize sleep by taking three steps:

- ✓ First, go to bed one hour earlier and rise one hour later to start. Shoot for 9 hours of sleep every night.
- ✓ Second, I want you to take a brief 10 to 20 minute nap between the hours of noon and 4:00 pm five days a week.
- ✓ Finally, I want you to meditate for 5 minutes by focusing on your breath at least 3 times per week.

Post-Menopause—Estrogen and Progesterone Deficient

At this point in your life, age has caused your ovaries to lose their ability to respond to the demands of your metabolism. That means that you need to learn how to anticipate those demands, and take action to respond.

The most important step you can take is to reduce stress, and for post-menopausal women sleep is the number one best stress reducer you can engage in. The irony is, you may find it harder to sleep now than you did in your younger years due to the changes in your hormone levels.

When sleep is problematic, naps and meditation work wonders. Research shows that even a 10 to 30 minute nap can undo many of the hormonal problems caused by sleep loss.[33] Meditation has also been shown to restore function in the body and brain similar to how a nap does.

I want you to prioritize sleep by taking three steps:

- ✓ First, go to bed one hour earlier and rise one hour later to start. Shoot for 9 hours of sleep every night.
- ✓ Second, I want you to take a brief 10 to 20 minute nap between the hours of noon and 4:00 pm five days a week.
- ✓ Finally, I want you to meditate for 5 minutes by focusing on your breath at least 3 times per week.

REST-BASED LIVING RECOMMENDATIONS FOR EVERYONE

Of course, your options for relaxation go way beyond those outlined for your specific hormone type. The solution to a stress-filled life lies in understanding that the fast-paced, get-it-done-now, never-take-a-break, harder-faster-longer mindset is the problem. Lifestyle choices matter. There are many choices you can make that lower stress hormones and help the metabolism get back into balance.

Connection Therapy

✓ Laughing lowers cortisol. This is why time with friends, connection to family, hanging with pets, and anything else that puts you in a happy mood is key.

✓ Sex and cuddling, both separately and more powerfully when combined, are powerful stress reducers.

✓ Orgasm, whether through masturbation or sex, immediately puts the metabolism in relax and recovery mode. Add a long cuddle to that and you are in stress-relieving bliss.

Water Therapy

✓ Long showers and relaxing baths are an excellent option.

✓ Relaxing spa-like music with candlelight is a perfect way to amplify the stress-relieving benefits of water therapy.

✓ Hot baths happen to be a wonderful way to detoxify your body, eliminating toxins through the sweat while relaxing. Sweating, in particular, may be especially beneficial to a subset of toxins called persistent organic pollutants or POPs. These compounds can act in the body as hormone disruptors and therefore their removal has the potential to rebalance hormone function.

Relaxation Therapy

✓ Get plenty of sleep. Sleep deprivation elevates stress hormone production and sends SHMEC out of check.

✓ Take naps. Research has shown that even a 10 minute nap can undo much of the dysfunction associated with sleep deprivation. And it is much better than adding in another work out.

✓ Get a massage. Massage has benefits due to its ability to focus the mind on the present, relax the metabolism and release muscular tension and strain.

✓ Even self-massage techniques like foam rolling are wonderful for stress.

✓ Practice meditation. The relative contribution of sympathetic (stimulation) and parasympathetic (relaxing) activity is balanced out. Mindfulness has also been shown to help those who practice it become more stress-resistant over time.

Movement Therapy

✓ Avoid heavy exercise. Pilates and exercise classes are typically not relaxing, so you don't need to do more than what is outlined in this program. If you want to integrate these kinds of activities into your daily plan, follow the steps to do this outlined in Chapter 8.

✓ The yoga of the Western world is typically intense and stimulating. Things like power yoga are not going to do the trick, but relaxing and stretching types of yoga are great.

✓ Tai chi is a wonderful option. This activity integrates mindfulness and slow rhythmic movements of the body. The outcome is very similar to walking in its ability to calm and center the metabolism.

✓ Take a walk. Take many walks. Walking lowers cortisol. It can't be huffing puffing, arm-swinging power walking that is more akin to running. This type of walking is slow and relaxing and allows you to take in the scenery. This is why walking is so central to this program.

The idea is to schedule these rest, recovery and relaxation sessions into your daily life as much as possible. Specifically, making walking the central focus of your stress reduction and then using other modalities daily or even multiple times per day are going to make all the difference in the world.

Find and use as many different tools and techniques as you can. The modern day provides increasing options in this regard. Spas, deprivation chambers, massage therapists, saunas, the list goes on and on.

The point is to find what works for you and do it. Use the techniques to decrease your stress output and your body will thank you. Do not neglect this portion of the program. It's one of the worst mistakes you can make for your body shape goals.

And, if you're "doing everything right" but still feel stuck, I hope this chapter helps you get unstuck in a way you may not even have realized was so important.

WHAT YOU LEARNED IN THIS CHAPTER:

- ✓ Chronic stress is devastating for your health and body shape. It forces your body to pile on fat, especially around the middle.
- ✓ Integrating rest-based living into your life is one of the most important things you can do for fat loss. It's more important than exercise, and maybe even more important than diet.
- ✓ So reducing your overall stress profile, by integrating daily relaxing activities into your program is crucial.
- ✓ Walking and other forms of non-exercise movement are essential. They are a key factor in the fat-loss equation and can help you relax as well.
- ✓ Do not skip this part of the program. It may be more important than everything else you have learned so far.

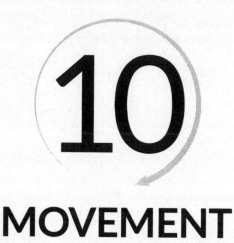

MOVEMENT

Most people don't understand why I would distinguish movement from metabolics. They wonder what the difference is between the two.

Exercise, or metabolics, is certainly a type of movement. It is a structured, planned event with the distinct goal of stimulating the metabolism for some defined goal. Burn fat, build muscle, get faster, get stronger or train longer.

Movement is just what you do when you are living. It is what you do when you walk down to the store, fidget, garden, clean the house, have sex or type on your computer. All that stuff is what researchers call non-exercise associated thermogenesis (NEAT).

It turns out this kind of movement is a huge component of total daily energy use. Research looking at a person who sits all day long and then does a 30-minute workout (metabolics) compared to a person who moves all day long but does not do structured exercise suggests that the mover is far better off health and fitness wise than the metabolic exerciser.[34,35]

This NEAT movement is also dramatically impacted by eating less and exercising more. The less you eat and the more you exercise, the more the body compensates by decreasing NEAT.

If you are not taking NEAT into account, then you are not doing everything right, no matter what you think. This is one of the reasons why policy makers suggest walking 10,000 steps per day. It is a way to make sure that we move more in the way that our naturally thin ancestors did.

Up until the 1960s the only people who exercised were athletes. Everyone else just carried on with the activities of daily living. And, surprisingly, these people were much leaner, fitter and healthier than we are today.

By all accounts, more people do structured exercise today than at any other time in the history of mankind, yet the modern day exercising man or woman is heavier than past generations.

At first this discrepancy may seem to make little sense until you look at the statistics on moving. Our ancestors moved all day every day. Research shows that our hunter-gatherer ancestors walked from 7 to 20 miles every day, often carrying babies and hauling gear in the process. In contrast, modern day men and women sit for 95% or more of their waking day.

This has profound implications on health.

WHY MOVING MORE MAY BE MORE IMPORTANT THAN EXERCISE

Recently a rash of research has shown that inactivity may be the biggest risk factor of all for diabetes and heart disease, two of the end-stage consequences of a damaged metabolism.

In one recent study published in the May 2013 issue of the journal *Diabetologia*,[36] researchers showed that movement was a far better predictor of health than either moderate or even intense physical exercise.

In other words, sitting all day long and then going for a vigorous 30 minute run was not nearly as effective for health and metabolic function as just moving more.

This research, and other studies like it, have led many experts in the health and fitness fields to begin focusing much of their efforts on getting people to move more rather than exercise more.

Some of the new recommendations coming out of this research hints that organizations such as the American Heart Association, the American Diabetes Association and the American College of Sports Medicine should set a daily limit on sitting time. Many believe this limit should be no more than 90 minutes.

I realize this information can be a little confusing, but once you think about it, it starts to make intuitive sense.

But can simply moving more really help with weight loss and be better than exercise?

A study in the October 2005 issue of the journal *Chest* showed that jogging for 12 miles a week was not much different than walking for 12 miles a week from a weight-loss perspective and that both dramatically enhanced cardiovascular health.[37]

You may be surprised by that finding, but when you consider that many studies have shown that intense exercise, while healthy, can cause compensatory reactions that increase hunger and cravings leading to food compensation, studies like these begin to make sense.

Some believe this effect is mediated by the stress hormone cortisol. Intense exercise releases more cortisol into the body, and this can have damaging effects. These effects seem to be mitigated by low-intensity movements like walking.

GO FOR A WALK

Walking allows you to move far more often without extra stress to your body and is one of the only forms of exercise that has been shown to lower cortisol and have a minimal impact on hunger. It also seems to be even more effective when done in a natural setting.

The take home is that more exercise is not really that beneficial, but more movement is. You would be better off moving all day than sitting all day and then doing an intense bout of exercise. Walking lowers cortisol and does not stimulate the appetite.

That is why I recommend you try to get at least 10,000 steps per day. This should be a major focus of your program. Even if you follow the meals and metabolics guidelines to a T, I can almost guarantee that you will not see the results you want if you don't walk. We are built to move. So do what you were made to do and get your steps in.

Keep in mind that 5,000 steps is a little less than an hour a day for most people. If you shoot for two hours of walking, you'll be golden. Don't worry, this is not two hours at one time. When I say two hours, this is just total accumulated time walking around. A better way to measure this is to use a step counter. Two hours is about 10,000 accumulated steps during the day.

ADJUSTING FOR YOUR HORMONE TYPE

Here are a few tips you can integrate based on your hormone type. These may help you take your movement a bit further.

Normal Menstrual Cycle—Estrogen and Progesterone Balanced

Given your more balanced and stable hormonal rhythms, you should be able to benefit from as much walking as you like. As long as the walking is slow and relaxed you really can't do too much.

In fact, this is one of the few places where more may be better. That being said, even walking can be overdone, so pay attention to changes in SHMEC to determine whether you are taking it too far.

Normal Menstrual Cycle—Estrogen Dominant

Given the extra estrogen you may be dealing with, you will want to shoot for the upper limit of walking. For you 10,000 steps a day should be a minimum, while 20,000 steps per day is probably the maximum you need. Try to keep your steps in this range.

Normal Menstrual Cycle—Progesterone Deficient

Because you are dealing with stress issues—one of the major causes of progesterone falling—you will want to make sure walking is done enough but not too much. Shoot for 10,000 steps per day at first. Then every few weeks you can increase the walking load by 1,000 to 2,000 steps per day. Just make sure you add steps slowly.

Normal Menstrual Cycle—Estrogen and Progesterone Deficient

The major thing impacting you is stress. You may be more sensitive to stress than perhaps any other hormonal type.

Remember, both estrogen and progesterone work together to keep a lid on the negative effects of cortisol. When both fall, it is not going to be a good thing for the way your body looks. This is one of the major causes of being normal weight but still dealing with belly fat issues.

You will want to use walking very carefully since for you it can be more easily overdone. Start with 5,000 steps per day and then slowly increase that by 5,000 steps per day each week. If SHMEC goes out of check, dial it back. Try to keep your walking to less than 20,000 steps per day.

You also may want to consider walking while listening to slow relaxing spa music to make sure you go slow and take your time. Walking in natural settings is even more beneficial.

Perimenopause—Estrogen Fluctuating, Progesterone Deficient

This is a volatile time where some days you will feel balanced and productive and other days you may feel crazy.

Walking a little faster and more briskly (somewhere between a slow walk and powerwalking, i.e., 3 to 4 mph) first thing in the morning when you wake up can have an energizing and balancing effect on your entire system. Reducing the speed at night to a slow meander while practicing deep breathing along with the walking can help with sleep and anxiety. Walking for you can be done whenever, but is best done morning and evening. Shoot for 10,000 steps per day.

Menopause—Estrogen and Progesterone Deficient

Now that you have made it through perimenopause, things are a lot less volatile. You can and should definitely ramp up your walking to between 10,000 and 20,000 steps per day, which means 2 to 4 hours daily. I realize this seems like a lot, but this can be accumulated in all daily activity. Walking around at work, laundry, gardening, etc.

To make your movement work best for you try to do two to three 30 to 40 minute walks throughout the day in addition to staying active and on your feet. Remember, SHMEC will guide you. Walking is hard for you to overdo and is one of the few things where more is almost always better. But sometimes it can be too much. If SHMEC is in check you are on the right path.

Post-Menopause—Estrogen and Progesterone Deficient

At this stage of life you are still dealing with low estrogen and progesterone, but also a higher relative level of testosterone. This may thicken and amplify the belly fat issues women dread. Walking is the belly fat killer, because it helps buffer against the insulin and cortisol effects induced by the loss of female hormones.

Shoot for 10,000 to 20,000 steps per day. You can do this through 2 two hour walks, four 1 hour walks, or just accumulate the steps through your general daily activities. To help count your steps, consider looking at an activity tracker.

And remember, this does not mean that exercise is not important. In fact, there may be a synergistic effect when walking is combined with intense exercise.

This is why I recommend a slow 30 minute walk after your workouts. While elevated cortisol is good and beneficial for fat-burning during exercise, it is not great for it to remain high after exercise.

Walking can immediately bring down cortisol after a workout. Doing your walk after your workout also gets you up and moving more without an exorbitant time investment. And it's just flat out enjoyable.

So make time to go for a walk after your workouts if you can, and don't forget to get up and move around more throughout your day. Walk to the market, take the stairs at work, go out for a gentle hike with your family, or do whatever else gets you up and moving more.

WHAT YOU LEARNED IN THIS CHAPTER:

- ✓ Movement is different than exercise.
- ✓ Moving all day and not exercising may be better than sitting still all day and then exercising.
- ✓ Walking mixed with intelligent metabolic-enhancing exercise may be the most powerful combination of all.
- ✓ While elevated cortisol is good and beneficial for fat burning during exercise it is not great to have high cortisol after exercise.
- ✓ Walking can immediately bring down cortisol after a workout.

HOW TO GET STARTED ON THE *METABOLIC RENEWAL* PROGRAM

M It is time to get started with the program, but before you do, I want to give you a brief overview and a few pointers.

MEALS

To get going on the meals plan, here is what to do:

- ✓ **Step 1: Select the diet that's right for you based on where you are in your life.** Menstruating women can cycle, menopausal women should stick to the ELEL approach.
- ✓ **Step 2: Optimize based on hormone type.** Add the tips I outlined for how to further optimize the meal plan based on your hormone type.
- ✓ **Step 3: Follow the AIM protocol.** Later on you can further personalize this program by tuning into SHMEC and adapting the diet to fit your unique metabolic needs.

Of course, there is one question I haven't answered, and that's what specific foods you should eat. That's because I have laid all of that out for you in your *12-Week Metabolic Renewal Meal Plan*. You have a few options on how to use that:

1. Follow the delicious menus and recipes in the *12-Week Metabolic Renewal Meal Plan*.
2. "Roll your own" meals using the guidelines for doing this in the meal plan.
3. Do some combination of the two.

Whatever you choose, all of the details are in the meal plan. We have included specific guidelines on what foods to eat, what foods not to eat, added some suggestions for snacks and additional meals if that applies to you, and more.

The recipes we have developed are not only spectacularly delicious, but we have kept them to the absolute highest nutritional standards we could. I'll tell you, it's not an easy task to create restaurant-quality meals that are still extremely healthy, but that is precisely what we have done with this program.

Basically, all of the work is done for you. Just select the nutrition plan based on where you are in your cycle or time of life, optimize it for your hormone type, check out the *12-Week Metabolic Renewal Meal Plan*, and then use the AIM process to fine-tune the diet to your personal needs.

If you did this—really followed the nutrition plan I have laid out in this program—and nothing else, you'd get results, and you'd change the whole way you think about food and dieting. You'd move from a dieter's mindset to that of a metabolic detective. Does that sound like something you're interested in?

It won't be easy… but I know you can do it. So what have you got to lose? Study your metabolism. Enjoy delicious food. And figure out what works for you.

METABOLICS (EXERCISE)

Everyone will start with the core *Metabolic Renewal* workouts on the videos that are included in your program. You will do these three times a week for 15 minutes. Then you can adapt this as follows:

✓ If you are a menstruating woman, you can add up to three additional workouts of your choosing during the follicular phase of your cycle when you shift to an EMEM approach.

✓ If you are a menopausal woman, you may need to dial this back and only do two workouts a week if SHMEC goes out of check.

And, of course, I added some additional tips for each hormone type.

A few things you should know about the *Metabolic Renewal* workouts:

These routines were designed in a specific sequence. There are four phases in total and each phase lasts for three weeks.

✓ **Phase 1 Harmonize:** Phase 1 gets your hormone-signaling systems working properly so you can enjoy the benefits of exercise without overloading you with too much stress. The simple moves gently restore your brain's "command and control center," which awakens your metabolism.

✓ **Phase 2 Inspire:** Now that you've awakened your metabolism and reset your hormones, Phase 2 will inspire your body's cellular machinery to burn body fat for fuel. A new set of moves wake up your cells and your mitochondria (your cellular energy factories) to turn fat into energy at top speed.

✓ **Phase 3 Enhance:** Your metabolism is humming, your hormones are in harmony, and your fat-burning machinery is firing… you're now ready to turn up the dial in Phase 3 with a new set of more intense movements. Without taking the steps you did in Phases 1 and 2, your body wouldn't be able to handle the increased fat-burning intensity for long, but now you can.

✓ **Phase 4 Symphony:** Now you can crank up the intensity dial to the fullest setting your body is ready for. This taps into the unique hormonal advantage that is the hallmark of the female metabolism: human growth hormone (HGH). The signature "burn" movements stimulate HGH, your primary metabolic multitasker, to tighten your belly, butt, hips and arms.

Each phase contains three different workouts—one workout for Monday, one for Wednesday and one for Friday. If the Monday, Wednesday and Friday schedule doesn't suit you, feel free to adjust to a Tuesday, Thursday and Saturday schedule or any other schedule that works for you. For best results, leave one day of recovery between workouts.

THE CRITICAL IMPORTANCE OF REST

It is important to remember that this style of training is different from the way most approach exercise. I *do not* want you to pace yourself in these workouts. You goal is to push yourself as hard as you can within your fitness level until you are forced to stop and rest. You then rest as long as is required to exert strong intensity once again.

The key point is that the whole workout is only 15 minutes, *INCLUDING* rest, and you should rest as much as you need to. Do *NOT* pause the video to rest, keep it going and just pick back up when you are ready. The 15 minutes is truly 15 minutes of elapsed time, which includes both your exercise and your rest time.

The most beneficial workouts will have you resting almost as frequently as you are working. Beginners may even find that they rest *more* than they work. Some people will naturally gravitate to longer rests that are less frequent and others will prefer shorter, more frequent rest periods. Whatever allows you to generate the greatest intensity is best.

Feel free to experiment based on your preferences, **but rest is essential**. Without rest, the workout quality will be compromised and you will revert back to a less efficient style of training.

The mantra to burn into your mind is "Push until you can't, rest until you can."

One final consideration on the exercises is to make sure you pay close attention to my cues during the workouts. For example, to get the most out of the squeezing exercises, you will need to stay focused. I'll help you. Do your best not to rush the exercises and really work on squeezing tight on the areas you are working.

If you keep these pointers in mind, you will get the most out of the workout.

The Burnout Session

I have also included a little something extra in the *Metabolic Renewal* workouts. The burnout session is a super-intense callisthenic and plyometric workout that is designed to accentuate the breathless component of the workout.

This does two beneficial things. It creates an even greater metabolic effect, but it also makes doubly sure that we can burn up all the fat that was released during the workout.

Just because stored fat is released from fat cells, that does not necessarily mean it will be burned; fat cells can suck it back in if the muscles don't burn it up for energy. The burnout session is extra insurance that your muscles can mop up all the fat that was mobilized from the main workout.

The best way to make sure this fat is burned and not restored is to put a little more demand on your metabolism at the end. You need to convince your body that it not only needs to burn the fat that is released, but do it quickly. But don't be worried. The truth is that the burnout session is not required. It is there for those who feel like they have a little extra in them, and love and want a different challenge.

And remember, as a woman your metabolism is a little more stress-reactive. Depending on where you are in your cycle or phase of life, these burnout sessions can either be just right or a little too much. Don't make the mistake of thinking more is always better.

Finishing with a Walk and Cool-Down

In reality, the best way to ensure that the workout has maximum benefit is to include a leisurely walk after the workout, if you have time. Unlike intense exercise, this walking will lower cortisol and stress hormones. While we want cortisol and catecholamines high during the workout, we want to shut them down when the workout is over. Leisurely walking is a great way to do this.

It's also a great way to get in your steps and fulfill the movement part of this program.

After the workout, a leisurely walk for 30 to 60 minutes is great. But you will get the benefits even if you do it for 5 to 10 minutes. Any little bit counts. Ideally, I'd like to see you walking one to two hours on all or most days of the week. If that isn't practical, do what you can. Always do your walking last and don't forget to stretch, too. I did not include a standard cool-down in the *Metabolic Renewal* workouts because I have found a lot of people do their own thing anyway. But if you want my number one recommendation for a post-workout cool-down, it's a leisurely walk.

MINDSET

To really produce benefits from the *Metabolic Renewal* program, you actually have to learn to do just that; renew. Diet and exercise are only 50% of the equation. The rest is about mindset and movement.

Your lifestyle should be constantly programming your body to handle stress better. There are so many different types of activities that optimize the metabolic process through reprogramming stress reactions. I call these rest and recovery activities and you should be shooting to include at least one of these activities per day. If you can't fit that many in, try for a bare minimum of three per week. I have provided specific recommendations for each hormone type as well as a bunch of others you can try if you want.

These activities include creative pursuits like writing, painting or other artistic activities. Meditation and mindfulness activities are a huge piece as well. Don't worry, it is not necessary to become a monk. Sitting quietly with herbal tea looking out the window watching the birds, listening to relaxing music, sitting quietly on a park bench watching the world go by, or reading a book, are all forms of mindfulness and meditation. Massage, spa therapies, hot baths and long showers all lower stress hormones.

One taboo topic of the Western world is sex and orgasm. For some reason, we get a little uncomfortable talking about it. It may be one of the most restorative and relaxing things you can do. Orgasm, whether through masturbation or sex, is one of the more enjoyable ways to maximize results in this program.

In fact, women compared to men have unique brain changes after orgasm that result in more focus, greater pain tolerance, and lower levels of stress hormones. It may be that due to changes in focus and pain reduction, that orgasms both before exercise and after may have benefits for women, where only after may benefit men.

Use all these activities to your advantage by scheduling, prioritizing and emphasizing them in your life. Unfortunately, TV and computer time don't seem to have the same relaxing effects, unless they are shows and media that make us laugh.

MOVEMENT

Daily movement is crucial. NEAT is now known to be a huge component in weight loss and health. Look for every opportunity to move. Exercise is often not enough to overcome a lifestyle that involves sitting all day every day.

When you can stand, stand. When you can move, move. Make a game out of it if possible. Investing in an activity tracker and seeking to accumulate 30,000 to 70,000 steps a week is a great start.

TRACKING YOUR RESULTS

Another critical part of this plan is tracking your results. Why is this so important? Well, there are several reasons and I explain them all in your *Metabolic Renewal Transformation Tracker.* But basically it comes down to this: We humans are capable of incredible delusion, and the only way to get around that is to have objective data and feedback. That is what tracking gives you.

I've seen this over and over again with clients. (Heck, I've even experienced it myself.) One day you may wake up feeling crappy and when you look in the mirror you think, 'I look fat as hell!" Then the next day you wake up on the right side of the bed and think, "I don't look that bad. In fact, I'm looking pretty hot." Psychology plays an enormous role in how we perceive our bodies.

Tracking takes psychology out of the equation and allows us to make choices about our diet and exercise habits based on objective data. Plus, tracking your results provides you immediate, highly motivating feedback on improvements that are actually happening underneath the hood, but that you can't quite see yet.

With *Metabolic Renewal* your body, mind and overall health will start to improve rapidly, so the more closely you track this process, the more positive feedback you'll receive and the more motivated you'll be to keep going. This is why I want you to track your results throughout this program. The day before you begin you will take your first measurements. Then each week over the course of the program you will track your results to see how much progress you have made.

And I'm not just talking about weighing yourself here. In fact, that is the absolute least important parameter I want you to track. I'm talking about checking in with yourself and seeing how your sleep, hunger, mood, energy and cravings (your SHMEC) are doing. I'm talking about tracking changes in your health, your body shape, your hourglass figure and more. All of the details are in your tracker. So, go check that out before you start the program as well.

Okay, let's get started. After you've reviewed the nutrition guide and taken your initial measurements, load up the first workout and get it on.

Don't worry. I will be there to guide you throughout. Good luck.

WHAT YOU LEARNED IN THIS CHAPTER:

✓ You can't out-train a bad diet, so make sure to work on your nutrition using the information I have provided for that.

✓ The *Metabolic Renewal* program is a 12-week, 4-phase system that contains 3 different workouts per week.

✓ You do each phase for three weeks, progressing from one to the next sequentially.

✓ After each workout you can complete the burnout session if you want to burn up a little more fat.

✓ My favorite cool-down is a leisurely walk, but you can also cool down with full-body stretching.

✓ Lifestyle changes—especially walking, relaxation and detoxification—are extremely important as well. So make sure you integrate those changes into your life.

✓ Tracking your results is one of the most important things you can do, as it takes psychology out of the equation, providing you with objective feedback and data.

WEIGHT-LOSS ACCELERATION PHASE (OPTIONAL)

Once you've been on *Metabolic Renewal* for 8 weeks, your body and metabolism should be primed and ready to take your fat loss efforts to the next level, should you deem that path right for you. In this section, you will learn how to both amplify and speed your fat-loss results.

Now I know you may be thinking, "But Jade, I thought the entire purpose of this program was to not be thinking about fast, unrealistic body change." That is true, but what I did not tell you before is that when the body is primed appropriately, it can respond in very big ways.

Your metabolism is now perfectly prepared to be stimulated for big time fat loss. Let me explain.

THE TRUTH ABOUT METABOLISM

One of the most important things you have learned is that the metabolism is not what you thought it was. It does not care about your vanity concerns, your timetables, or whether things are convenient for you or not. This is a point you must never forget.

The metabolism is an adaptive-reactive system that thrives in an environment where food intake and exercise output are more closely aligned. This is why the eat less/exercise less (ELEL), and eat more/ exercise more (EMEM) protocols work so well. Add to this the cyclical approach to dieting you have now learned, and you can greatly amplify your results.

I hope these concepts are seared into your subconscious by now, so you never again will make the mistake of following the old way as a long-term strategy.

The old way, of eat less and exercise more (ELEM) is only effective for a short period of time. It is too stressful for the metabolism to maintain for long. That being said, when the metabolism is healthy and primed, both the eat less/exercise more protocol (ELEM) and the eat more/exercise less protocol (EMEL) can provide some benefit.

The reason they backfire on almost everyone is due to one simple fact: That is all people know and so that is all they do.

However, you have now learned that there are four distinct metabolic toggles. Two of these toggles should be used only for short periods of time (ELEM and EMEL). Two of these protocols can be used for much, much longer periods of time, perhaps even as a lifelong approach depending on the person (EMEM and ELEL).

My rule of thumb based on my clinical experience is that EMEM and ELEL can be used for months before any metabolic compensation kicks in. In some people, these protocols never result in metabolic compensation and thus can be followed for life.

Eat more and exercise less (i.e., EMEL, the couch-potato approach) can be very useful if done for a very short period of time. Usually this approach will start causing issues within 2 to 7 days. This is why I don't typically recommend anyone take this approach for more than a week or two weeks at the most. When limited to a very brief period (e.g., the holiday period or vacations are my two favorites), this can be beneficial in the context of an otherwise balanced ELEL or EMEM approach.

The eat less/exercise more (ELEM) model can be pushed for a little bit longer. Most people will begin to compensate on this approach after 10 to 14 days. Some can go longer, but virtually everyone will start seeing negative metabolic effects after 4 weeks of this approach.

But here is the beautiful thing for you. Your metabolism has now had 8 weeks to reprogram and restore some of the flexibility it lost. This newfound metabolic power means going back to an EMEL approach for a short time will result in less fat storage and more metabolic benefits.

IT'S HOW OUR ANCESTORS LIVED AND ATE

Imagine a historical female hunter-gatherer who has been moving day in and day out and eating adequately throughout the summer. Or perhaps she is just coming out of late winter or early spring. Food has been sparse and she has been on the move relentlessly to supply herself and her tribe with food. Perhaps she and her tribe then make a particularly rewarding hunt-and-gather session. They have enough food for everyone to eat heartily for the next few weeks.

At that point, her metabolism's natural intelligence will cause her to eat, rest and recover. In this context, EMEL is not only healthy, but also will aid lean tissue and help her stay fit and functional. Of course, in the natural world, it would be virtually impossible for this condition to endure beyond a few days or a few weeks.

Eat less, exercise more (ELEM) can be very beneficial as well in the right context and when the metabolism is primed for it. Think about the female hunter living with her tribe in natural settings. She will likely spend the summer and early fall in more of an eat more/exercise more approach (EMEM). She will then likely have a middle to late fall with plenty of foods, fruits and fatty animals storing up for the winter months.

She may encounter an EMEL state more often than normal. But that is useful because winter is coming and will almost certainly result in spending time in an eat less / exercise less (ELEL) state.

Then early spring comes. Animals are lean. Fruits and vegetables are slim pickings. She is forced for a short time to be in an eat less/exercise more state (ELEM). This won't last too long though, as she will slowly drift back into plenty of food and plenty of movement.

APPLYING THE WISDOM OF NATURE

This type of seasonal cyclical approach is an amazing way to continue to keep the metabolism healthy and get extra lean.

So, after 8 weeks on the program, we are going to purposely expose your female metabolism to this eat less/exercise more approach (ELEM). At this point, not only can your body handle it, but it becomes an amazing way to amplify your results.

But remember that this is a very tricky time. You do not want to make the mistake everyone else makes and take this to the extreme of doing it for too long. SHMEC must always continue to guide you.

You must realize the only reason this is going to work is because of the ELEL and EMEM approach you have been following. Without this context, ELEM will likely backfire, giving you short-term results and then long-term weight gain.

So, as we purposely begin to move in the ELEM approach, you must keep two things in mind. First, realize that this is temporary and can, depending on your unique metabolism, cause serious imbalances in your metabolism. This will vary and SHMEC will tell you. If this happens, then you move back to a more balancing EMEM or ELEL until you feel stable enough to try again.

Second, this **should only be done for 4 weeks at the longest**, even if you feel great the entire time. Going to extremes or continuing the regimen too long with any dietary regime will, without a doubt, backfire on you.

So, I want you to agree with me right here that you will not fall back into old patterns and start becoming the dieter again. Remember, this is about leaving that dieting mentality behind. You cannot follow one-size-fits-all meal plans, food lists and recipes and expect that they will not become a crutch.

The idea is to follow the axiom that one of my heroes, Bruce Lee, advocated, "absorb what is useful, discard what is not and add what is uniquely your own."

This is the way it works. You don't find a diet; you create a lifestyle. The faster you learn that, the better off you will be.

And believe it or not, that is the real reason I want you to switch gears this last 4 weeks. I want to see if you have gotten what I wanted you to get. If you don't get the practice now, then what's going to happen when you get out in the "real world."

To refine your metabolic detective skills, you need to expose your metabolism to things that may be challenging for it and then learn to adjust and react. There is no way you are going to be able to accomplish complete body change and make it last in 12 weeks.

But, do that 12 weeks properly, by learning a process rather than following a protocol, and you can grow, learn, and get better over time. That is the exact opposite of what happens in most other approaches, isn't it?

So we are going to give you some real-world practice now by switching you into an eat less/exercise more approach (ELEM). Why? Because I want you to see that there is nothing wrong about this approach. In fact, done the right way, in the right context, with a flexible metabolism, it can be a great way to make progress as long as you don't go too far.

WHAT TO EAT LESS OF?

When it comes to eating less, there are a lot of things you could eat less of. We could focus on carbs. We could focus on fat. Or we could focus on calories. In truth, if you reduce any food group without increasing others you will be automatically decreasing calories.

And that's what we really want. We want to give your new, more flexible metabolism a challenge by widening the gap between food intake and energy output.

This will do several things. For a short period of time, the body will be forced to supply itself with energy because of this greater caloric deficit. This will hopefully result in speeding up fat loss.

Of course, you have learned that this will only last a short time before the body starts to throw SHMEC out of check and purposely slow its fat loss to compensate. But if we take this approach consciously for a short period of time, we can burn some extra fat and be back in a balanced EMEM or ELEL approach before the metabolism knows what hit it.

I am going to suggest that we cut carbohydrates instead of fat. I also think this works better than just indiscriminately cutting calories down. But please, don't jump to the conclusion that we are cutting carbs because they are "bad" or a "fat-storing food." In reality, that is a completely false idea and not helpful for you in your long-term journey.

I like cutting carbs for several reasons. One reason is that carbs are widely available and the easiest food group to get access too. I like focusing on cutting back on carbs because it helps you practice being more mindful of all the places they show up.

I also like to focus on carbs because carbohydrates increase your storage of glycogen in the liver and muscle. This stored sugar acts like a biological sponge soaking up about 2-3 times its weight in water.

This means that you will see a pretty big reduction in water weight when you cut carbs. When you add them back, you will see a similar rise in body weight. I want you to experience this so you can understand that a lot of the "miracle weight-loss" diets out there that taught "low-carb magic" are nothing but a method of creating this water effect.

You can use this "water effect" to look better for a short time, but it is not fat and it won't last. I want you to understand this and get used to the idea that wild, extreme fluctuations in weight are only water, and will almost always be transitory. This is very useful to know since it saves you from being duped by the low-carb advocates. It will also help you learn to obsess less about food as you learn that these water fluctuations are normal.

Finally, carbs and protein are both powerful stimulators of the hormone insulin. Insulin, when it is functioning correctly, is a great hormone. It helps us feel full. It helps us build muscle and it helps to make sure we can store extra calories in times of excess.

Because many people come from a standard western diet, they eat a very carb- and protein-heavy diet. This combination causes the body to produce too much insulin, which then leads to insulin dysfunction.

By cutting down on carbs, but leaving protein the same, we can continue to benefit from the hunger suppression of adequate protein while reducing some of the insulin production by trimming carbs. This can help us restore insulin's function and feel full for longer after meals. We also store less fat.

So, for this next 4 weeks, I want to take a one-size-fits-all approach of reducing your total carb intake (fiber included) to between 100 and 120 grams per day.

That word "one-size-fits-all" should make your eyebrows go up. You have already learned that this is the exact wrong approach. So, of course, you are going to adjust and we are going to use the structured flexibility approach.

We start with this low-carb intake without changing anything else. This will immediately put you in an eat less/exercise more (ELEM) state without doing anything with your exercise.

From there, you do what you have learned. You monitor SHMEC and results. If SHMEC goes out of check, you adjust by following the 5-step AIM process you have already learned.

In this way, we force the metabolism to deal with fewer carbs, and then we get to watch with keen interest how it responds. Then we adjust by first adding more protein, fiber and water-based foods. If that does not correct the SHMEC issues, we add fat. If that does not work, we follow the rest of the 5 steps.

And if things go really sideways, you always have ELEL or EMEM as your home base to return to, right? By now, you know which of these two approaches produces the most stability.

I realize that the idea of counting and weighing food is daunting. In truth, I don't want you to count at all. I have a very simple way for you to "count" without doing any math at all.

Here is the way to really think about this. Open up your hand and look at your palm. Now imagine a small measure of rice about the size of a large scoop of ice cream sitting in your palm. This serving of starch will cover your palm and be about 1 to 2 inches high. A serving of starch such as this will have about 30g of carbohydrate in it. This is also the rough equivalent of one cup of cooked rice, boiled potato or boiled pasta. It is the size of a small potato or a large piece of fruit.

All you need to do is limit yourself to three small handfuls of starchy foods per day. Each of these handfuls will represent about 30g or 120 calories per day.

In addition, you will not want to consume any packaged or processed foods that contain any more than 10g of carbohydrates after subtracting out the fiber.

This allows you to be able to easily reach this low level of carbohydrate intake without needing to count calories or measure grams of food.

So, that's it. No more than three small handfuls of starchy food (including all fruits) per day. Limit your packaged food intake to one serving only of foods containing 10g or less of carbs after subtracting out the fiber.

In case you are wondering which foods are considered starches and fruits, here is a small list: potatoes, sweet potatoes, all squashes (yellow, zucchini, spaghetti squash, etc.), rice, oats, quinoa, corn, beans, all fruits, pasta, breads and all boxed and packaged foods.

In addition, do not try to add on fat or protein to account for this drop in starchy foods. Simply reduce the starch intake and make no other food changes up or down.

Some may wonder, "But Jade, what if I am already eating very low levels of carbs?" For example, what if you are already eating less than 120g of total carbohydrates?

In this case, I want you to cut the current amount you are eating in half. Let's say your total carbohydrate intake is 75g. Take half of that and now you are consuming about 37g per day of carbohydrates.

Does that make sense? Super simple, right?

I am very excited for you to tackle this last 4 weeks. You now have all the tools necessary to make this 4 weeks productive and solidify your metabolic detective credentials.

Just remember, we are purposely exposing you to this to give you practice living this new lifestyle. Consider this as your graduation, and now you are doing your internship.

Let's get after it.

WHAT YOU LEARNED IN THIS CHAPTER:

✓ An eat-less-exercise-less (ELEL) approach can work if your metabolism is primed for it.

✓ After 8 weeks on this program, you should be ready to start leaning on your metabolism with an ELEL diet.

✓ Do this for only four weeks.

✓ Cut carbs down to 100 to 120 grams a day or half of what you are currently eating if it's less than that.

MOST FREQUENTLY ASKED QUESTIONS

I know some of you will have questions that have not been answered, so in this chapter I wanted to address the most frequently asked questions I get in my clinic. Scan through them and see if any apply to you. Or you can just move onto the next chapter if you are ready.

Do you have any tips for managing menstrual symptoms?

If you are in menses and experiencing symptoms like cramping, breast tenderness and other physical symptoms, you may want to consider a couple of supplements.

The first is krill oil, which I view as almost a female-specific essential fat. It's good for men too, but it seems to have an especially nice effect on women. There's a good study on PMS and krill oil consumption showing that women who take krill oil suffer from fewer symptoms.[38] I recommend trying one to three grams of krill oil daily. This may help allay some of your menstrual symptoms.

I also like the compound Vitex. Its common name is chasteberry. Between 400 and 800

milligrams per day is a really nice hypothalamus-pituitary-ovarian axis promoter. It balances the hypothalamus and can allay some of your symptoms. Note that it takes about four to eight weeks to begin seeing the effects of Vitex.

What if I am on birth control? Will that impact my program?

The important point to understand here is that contraceptives have synthetic hormones in them that bind more strongly to certain estrogen and progesterone receptors and more weakly to others.

The research is mixed, but it leans toward oral contraceptives speeding up the metabolism. Now, you might think this would be a good thing, but it typically results in SHMEC going out of check as well. As a result, many women hold more water and also end up having their hunger, energy, and cravings go out of check when they are on birth control. That's part of why they gain weight. This is not necessarily something that the hormones themselves are doing. The issue is that they can trigger changes in SHMEC.

The good news: By following the program, and keeping your SHMEC in check, you should be able to get the benefits of the oral contraceptive without the negative effects.

I'm on hormone replacement therapy. Is there anything I should be aware of?

There's two types of hormone replacement therapy (HRT), synthetic and bio-identical, and they are slightly different. The synthetic hormones bind to the estrogen and progesterone receptors more strongly in some tissues and more weakly in others. They're not exactly equivalent to natural estrogen and progesterone in the human body. So their effects can vary with different women.

The research on HRT suggests that they may have a slight weight-gain effect. However, they also seem to have a waist-slimming effect. That means women who are on HRT tend to maintain their hourglass shape a little bit better, but might end up getting a little heavier in the process. This is largely related to the fact that HRT will raise metabolic rate, which most people think is a good thing, but the metabolism compensates and can cause some women to eat more.

If you are on HRT, you can be happy with the idea that you're more likely to maintain your hourglass shape. You'll also probably have less signs and symptoms of menopause. But you have to be even more diligent with your diet than other people will need to be. Watch out for hidden increases in caloric consumption—particularly carbs—because this is bound to send SHMEC out of check and stall your fat loss attempts.

My bias is toward bio-identical hormone replacement, because they are bio-identical, and so behave the same as the estrogen and progesterone you make in your own body. The problem is that most prescription bio-identical hormones don't cycle like they do in a normally menstruating woman. The result is that you don't get the same results as you do with your naturally occurring hormones that fluctuate month to month. But they can definitely help for some, are better than synthetics in my opinion, and are nothing to be afraid of if your doctor recommends them. Just pay careful attention to SHMEC, follow the program, and you will be fine.

My doctor wants to put me on hormone replacement therapy. What do you recommend?

There's nothing wrong with going on HRT, especially when you consider that many women who are good candidates for it are suffering pretty dramatically with signs and symptoms that may keep them from working out or eating appropriately. HRT is not something to be afraid of. When possible, my bias is to use bio-identicals.

One thing to be aware if you are starting out on hormone replacement is that estrogen has a special relationship to thyroid hormone. If estrogen levels are too high, it can make thyroid hormone less effective. This has to do with how it changes the proteins that carry thyroid hormone around the body.

I suggest being screened for any thyroid-related issues before going on HRT. If you have low thyroid function you may want to have your thyroid closely monitored when you go on HRT.

Since this program affects hormones will it impact my ability to get pregnant?

This program will typically aid the healing of the metabolism. That's what we're trying to do. When the female metabolism is healed, it's more likely to sense that it's safe to carry a baby. So, oftentimes in my clinical experience, women who lose weight and optimize metabolic function actually have an easier time getting pregnant.

I am pregnant. To what extent can I do this program?

Research has come a long way in this area, and it now shows us that women who stay active through pregnancy usually have better pregnancy outcomes. However, there are a couple of things to think about as you start the program.

First, if you have never exercised intensely before, pregnancy is probably not the time to start. In that case, you may want to wait until baby arrives to begin the exercise portion of the plan. You can start all the rest right away. There aren't many (if any in this plan), but you may want to avoid any ballistic, jumping movements during the first trimester of your pregnancy. I also wouldn't suggest lots of running, pounding or jostling of the abdominal organs. It's a small risk, but it does exist. So you should know. In the third trimester, you should avoid doing lots of crunches or similar movements. Of course that is common sense, but worth mentioning.

With those caveats, this program is going to be very beneficial for most pregnant women. Of course, you should check with your physician and discuss the suitability of doing this program in your specific circumstance.

I have a preexisting medical condition. Is that going to impact the program?

It's beyond the scope of this program to address every individual case or medical condition out there. Rely on the judgment of your personal physician. And be aware that research shows that diet, exercise and lifestyle changes are among the most reliable healing modalities when it comes to all causes of morbidity and mortality.

By changing your lifestyle, you're doing a tremendous amount of good.

Will this program affect my libido?

Female libido is a little bit different than male. Women are more stress reactive. Women who are stressed out are going to see a drop in libido. That makes the rest-based living portion of this program even more important. Now in the context of exercise, metabolic dysfunction and libido, both eating less and exercising more will cause problems with libido because the body says, "Well, there's not enough resources to produce a baby."

Being overweight also is a stress on the body, so the body says, "Yeah, it's not really conducive to producing a baby." That means being overweight can also cause your libido to suffer.

This particular program balances the hypothalamus-pituitary-ovarian axis, adrenal axis and thyroid axis. That means it is basically optimizing female sexuality as well. You should not be surprised by an increased drive for both desire and performance sexually.

I am sick. Should I keep doing the program?

If you have a cold or flu that is just affecting your upper respiratory tract, you're safe to do exercise. If it's in the lungs or you have a fever, you want to stay in bed and take time off for your body to heal.

One thing that can be highly beneficial and help aid recovery from a cold or a flu—as well as provide some of the benefits of movement—is a hot hyperthermia bath. Pour a bath as hot as you can stand it.

Add four cups of Epsom salts optionally. Soak in the tub until it gets too uncomfortable to stay in. Then get out and wrap yourself up in sheets and blankets, get in bed and sweat.

The heat will increase blood flow throughout the body, giving you somewhat of a metabolic stimulus. Also, viruses and bacteria do not like hot environments. It's one of the reasons why our body mounts a fever in response to infection. So this will often delay or decrease the duration of a cold or a flu. Plus you get some of the benefits of exercise.

When you have a cold or the flu that's bad, it's a great opportunity to give your body good quality healing. Don't make the mistake that most people make and decide it's time to eat a bunch of junk food. Instead, consider illness is an opportunity for a metabolic reset. Feed your body correctly, with nourishing foods that are easy on the digestion like chicken soup. One supplement you can use when you're sick to support your immune system is glutamine powder. Glutamine is a fuel for the immune system. We use anywhere from 5 to 20 grams per day of powdered glutamine clinically.

If you have to take a break from exercise there's nothing wrong with just picking right back up where you left off if it's only been a week or two. But if it's been longer than that, you should start from the beginning.

I've fallen off the wagon. What's the best way for me to get back going on the program?

You're going to fall off the wagon sometimes. It's just something life does to all of us. The thing to do is to take it as a learning opportunity.

The number one thing I want to teach you in this program is that there is no wagon. There is just life happening. The more you can learn the skill of just starting back up when you fall off, the more you will make this into a lifestyle that fits your needs.

Don't tell yourself, "I'll start on Monday." Just start again, right now. There's no reason not to. Go back to the 3-2-1 Diet and work the program. Watch the videos and work out. Re-engage in rest-based living. Easy is earned. Nobody gets good at this overnight. Success comes with starts and stops, successes and failures, ups and downs, and plateaus and valleys.

You should assume you're going to have some mess-ups, missteps and setbacks along the way. That's life. It's the same with any program. The more you can get out of the mindset of, "Oh, I failed, and now I've got to start over," and instead think, "Okay, good, I knew this was going to happen, this is life, I'll just pick up right where I left off," the higher chance that this is going to become a lifestyle for you.

What if I don't get the results I want?

Typically when someone's not getting results it's almost always a result of not understanding the four major pillars of body change—movement, meals, metabolics and mindset. And usually when people aren't getting results, it's usually because they're putting too much emphasis on metabolics and meals and not enough emphasis on movement and mindset.

That means you need to pay closer attention to rest-based living and your basic daily movement—walking and things like that. Remember, non-exercise associated thermogenesis (NEAT) is the number one thing that we can do to create a sustainable calorie deficit. Most people want to "eat less, exercise more," or go on a detox, or something like that. If you aren't getting the results you want, I can almost guarantee this won't work.

The real thing you should be focusing on is more daily movement through walking and more rest-based living. The other thing I would say is this: If you're not getting results, then you're not eating and exercising the right way for you. You have to play metabolic detective. And when you do, it's not a matter of if, it's a matter of when.

The truth of the matter is that some people's metabolism requires far more walking, meal planning, and so on than others. Your metabolism doesn't particularly care that it is inconvenient for you to make these changes. So keep playing metabolic detective, and try to be patient and stay disciplined with the process.

Can I speed up my results even more?

Anytime you try to speed up results, you should remember that the metabolism is very much like a boomerang. Trying to push on it harder is going to make it push on you harder. So it's a big mistake to think about speeding things up.

A better question is: "How do I maintain nice, slow, steady weight loss and learn the skills I need to make it last?" That's going to come from building a base of movement and rest-based living, because those things together are restorative and healing for the metabolism and keep it revved up, whereas constantly focusing on diet and exercise can lead to issues.

WHAT HAPPENS WHEN THE 12 WEEKS ARE OVER?

After going through *Metabolic Renewal* you will likely emerge feeling stronger and leaner than you have in a very long time. This is a great place to be and is highly motivating. It's also a place where many people fall off the wagon.

Humans are weird. Once we find something that works, all of a sudden we want to change it. I see it in my clinic all the time. People see results, then they think they are done with the program and it's time to change to something else. This is exactly the wrong approach.

What you want to do is continue to work with your metabolism to make it even stronger, tighter and leaner. Ultimately that means challenging the metabolism. It's a little like math. Once you learn basic arithmetic you go into geometry and algebra. Eventually you even get to trigonometry and calculus.

You want to keep progressing this way physically as well. That ultimately means three things:

1. More weights
2. Higher intensity
3. Watching your SHMEC and altering your diet and lifestyle to fit these changes in weight and intensity

Here's what I recommend:

STEP 1: REPEAT THE ENTIRE 12-WEEK SEQUENCE AT LEAST 3 TIMES

Given the way these workouts are structured, you can and should turn right around and start the sequence again. That means doing the exact same version you just did (body weights, bands or dumbbells) again.

This time you will be more fit and more accustomed to the workouts. This time you'll know what's coming and you can focus on pushing yourself hard as follows:

1. **Squeezing Harder** – The squeezing movements are deceptively powerful but when you really squeeze hard, it's extraordinarily taxing and really stimulates your metabolism to become even more powerful, so on your next round try squeezing even harder on those movements.

2. **Increase Speed** – I never want you to go so fast that it sacrifices your form but increasing your speed while maintaining correct form can be a fantastic way to boost the intensity of your workout. Just try to progress through each move faster while keeping your form solid and you'll be able to complete more cycles of each movement in each round and set your metabolic fire ablaze. Remember, because this will tire you out even more quickly, you may need to rest more, which is fine.

3. **Burnout Sessions** – If you didn't do the burnout sessions your first time around, you can kick things up to the next level by giving them a try. When you are done with those, all four of the Bs and Hs will be cranking and you'll have created an absolute metabolic fat-burning inferno inside your body.

Once you have repeated the 12-week session you are doing 3 times (that means doing it for an entire year), you can move on to the next level of difficulty. For those of you who are starting out with the body weight versions of the exercises, that means you will do it with body weight alone 4 times (one year), then with bands 4 times (one year), then with dumbbells 4 times (one year).

If you think about it, this means you have 3 years of state-of-the-art metabolism rehabilitating exercise in this program alone.

STEP 2: KEEP AIM-ING FOR GOOD NUTRITION

As you make these changes in weight and intensity, make sure to continue monitoring your SHMEC. If it goes out of check, you may need to alter your diet and lifestyle to fit this new way of exercising. Remember, your metabolism is constantly adjusting. So if you press on it one way—by increasing the intensity of your exercise, for example—it's likely to push back in a different way. That means you may find you are more hungry, grumpy, tired, you crave foods you didn't, and so on.

You know what to do when this happens. Just go back to the AIM process, and figure out how to change your diet to fit the new demands on your body. You may need a little more starch or fat. Or maybe you need a little more fiber. Work the process.

STEP 3: MONITOR YOUR HORMONES AND ADJUST

Periodically you should also retake the Hormone-Type Quiz to check in with where you are. Remember, you can take that online at http://www.metabolicrenewal.com/quiz.

Your hormone balance can and will change as you integrate all of the steps in this program, restore, rebalance and renew your body from head to toe. Going back to the Hormone Type Quiz will help you continue to modify and optimize this plan for your ever-changing metabolism.

However, there are a few things to remember as you do this:

First, don't get so stuck in the idea of a "hormone type" that you start taking that idea as law. Your metabolism is uniquely your own. The Hormone-Type Quiz is just a place for you to see how things are progressing for you.

SHMEC should always be your real guide. Tune in to what is going on for you with your body. How do changes in the 4Ms impact SHMEC for you? What happens when you get super stressed out? Tune in and become that metabolic detective so you can always have a program that suits your particular needs.

Of course, when you hit post-menopause these fluctuations will dramatically decrease and your hormone type won't change all that much. That means you need to rely on SHMEC and the wisdom of your body and brain that much more. By this time in life, you'll have gained enough of that wisdom so you should be able to do this more effectively.

ENJOY YOUR LIFE!

Also pay attention to how to how much you are walking, resting and detoxifying. This is another area where we humans get funny. We suddenly think it's okay to stop doing activities that rejuvenate us. Don't do that. After all, life is short. Make it count. Do things that make you feel happy, relaxed and at peace. Why wouldn't you? Are your "responsibilities" really so important you can't take some time for yourself?

Assuming you repeat the program increasing intensity as you go, find a diet that works for your body using the AIM approach, and give your spirit the gift of rest and relaxation, I can almost guarantee you will be in the best shape of your life. At that stage, you might consider changing up the program a bit. You could try one of our other programs: *Metabolic Aftershock* or *Metabolic Prime*, for example.

On the other hand, those program may have been your way into this one, and that's fine too. You'll notice that there are nuances in each of these different programs. The diet is a little different. Some don't focus as much on lifestyle. This is partially by design, and it's partially just the nature of this business.

The fact is that I can't provide the perfect program for every single person on the planet. That just isn't possible. So every one of these programs is meant to be a set of guidelines you take and adapt to fit your personal needs.

If *Metabolic Prime* worked for you, and you want to try this *Metabolic Renewal* program and see how nutrition cycling works, go for it. On the other hand, if you've done *Metabolic Renewal* several times and you want to try some other workouts, switch it up with *Metabolic Aftershock* or *Metabolic Prime*. But when you do, always remember this: Study how your body reacts and adapts to the nuances built into these plans.

A lot of people have a tendency to "program hop" and think, "Oh, I'm done with this program, now I'll do that one." Don't do that. Investigate how each of these different plans works for you. It's not about changing all the time. It's about creating, rather than finding, the right diet, exercise and lifestyle plan for you. That will change over time and is always a work in process. You'll lose weight, burn fat, get more fit—and you'll need to adapt to that. You'll also get older, go through menopause, and need to adapt to that too.

The key is to react and adapt, just like your metabolism does, not by program hopping, but by continuing to work with your metabolism to seek the best solution for your personal needs. If there is one message I want you to take away from this program, that would be it. Don't keep looking for the next best thing on TV or the Internet. Create what works for you and keep doing that. Become a metabolic detective and leave the dieter's mindset behind once and for all. You won't regret it.

And I'll be here to support you every step of the way. Good luck!

WHAT YOU LEARNED IN THIS CHAPTER:

✓ When the 12-week program is over, repeat it 4 times and enhance the workout by squeezing harder, increasing your speed, and integrating the burnout sessions.

✓ Then you can progress to the next level and repeat that cycle 4 times.

✓ Assuming you are starting with the body weight exercises that means you have 3 years of workout routines in this program.

✓ Continue to AIM for good nutrition as you alter your exercise intensity.

✓ And make sure you are continuing your walking, relaxation and detoxification routines.

✓ Most of all, learn how to become a metabolic detective and leave the dieter's mindset behind once and for all.

CONCLUSION

Well, that's it. You have just completed reading through another program and have likely been following the *Metabolic Renewal* workouts for several days or even weeks.

At this point I want you to think about a few things. I want you to reflect on all the times in your past when you have started and completed a program. Or maybe you started and never finished.

What I want you to understand is that starting something is one of the easiest things you can do in this process. Finishing, of course, is much harder. But the idea of a finish line at least makes the hard work a little easier, right? Everyone loves having an end in sight.

That is what I want you to think about. In what other endeavor could you possibly spend only 8-12 weeks and expect to be a master at it? If you wanted to be a great pianist you would be working at it for years. If you wanted to learn to speak another language fluently, again, you would be at it for years. If you wanted to become a master chef it would require hours and hours and hours of cooking.

That is the way of the world. The path to mastery is not easy. And why would we expect it to be or even want it to be?

Nothing is easy. Easy is something you earn. It is something you figure out. Easy is a process of failure, discomfort, discovery, getting knocked down and getting up again.

In fact, if you asked anybody who is a master at their craft, "When did you reach the finish line?" Or, "How long did it take?" They would likely be confused or annoyed with the questions.

People who master a thing, don't look for a finish line and never consider themselves done. They don't want to be done. They have fallen in love with the process. It is part of who they are. It is what they love, and they relish the journey.

Why am I telling you this? Because I am incredibly excited for you. For your results. For the changes you will experience. For all the amazing benefits of a new body, revitalized metabolism and renewed health.

But I am also a little worried, because I know there is always the temptation to jump to the next new thing and forget what you have learned. It's just human nature. I am susceptible to it as well.

Just remember this: there is nothing wrong with trying new things. In fact, as a metabolic detective that can be very beneficial. But you must know how to do it correctly.

The famous martial artist, philosopher, and actor Bruce Lee describes the process perfectly. When it came to learning anything new he said we must, "absorb what is useful, discard what is not and add what is uniquely our own." This is the exact way I want you to view your body change and health endeavors from this moment on.

As you wrap up this experience you will no doubt be exposed to all kinds of new information. It will be a constant barrage. "Don't eat this," "Never eat that," "This is good," and "That is bad."

By now you should know to avoid paying too much attention to all of this noise. Your job—your only job—is to do what works for you. What works for you is different than what works for someone else. You are a woman, not a man. You are a unique woman with a metabolic expression as individual as your fingerprint, a psychology that is nuanced, and personal preferences you must honor.

When you get confused, curious or overwhelmed remember the process is where to point your effort. Always follow the process over any protocols. Structured flexibility, remember?

Start with any new thing you want to do, but then pay attention SHMEC and keep it in check.

If SHMEC is check, you're are burning fat (or maintaining your lean physique). If your vitals and blood labs are in a healthy range, then whatever you are doing is right for you.

This is the only way it works. It is the only way it has ever worked. You must continually build a diet and lifestyle uniquely suited to you—one built by you and for you.

I wish you much luck and continued success.

With gratitude,

Dr. Jade Teta

REFERENCES

[1] Trexler, Eric T., Abbie E. Smith-Ryan, and Layne E. Norton. "Metabolic adaptation to weight loss: implications for the athlete." *Journal of the International Society of Sports Nutrition* 11.1 (2014): 7.

[2] Levine, James A., et al. "Non-exercise activity thermogenesis." *Arteriosclerosis, thrombosis, and vascular biology* 26.4 (2006): 729-736.

[3] Wisløff, Ulrik, et al. "Superior cardiovascular effect of aerobic interval training versus moderate continuous training in heart failure patients a randomized study." *Circulation* 115.24 (2007): 3086-3094.

[4] Toohey K, Pumpa KL, Arnolda L, Cooke J, Yip D, Craft P, Semple S. "A pilot study examining the effects of low-volume high-intensity interval training and continuous low to moderate intensity training on quality of life, functional capacity and cardiovascular risk factors in cancer survivors." *PeerJ.* 2016 Oct 20;4:e2613. eCollection 2016.

[5] Sophie Cassidy, Christian Thoma, Kate Hallsworth, Jehill Parikh, Kieren G. Hollingsworth, Roy Taylor, Djordje G. Jakovljevic, Michael I. Trenell . "High intensity intermittent exercise improves cardiac structure and function and reduces liver fat in patients with type 2 diabetes: a randomised controlled trial." *Diabetologia* (2016) 59:56–66

[6] Joffrey Drigny. "Effect of interval training on cognitive functionING and cerebral oxygenation in obese patients: a pilot study." *J Rehabil Med* 2014; 46: 1050–1054.

[7] Morton SK, Whitehead JR, Brinkert RH, Caine DJ. (2011). "Resistance training vs. static stretching: effects on flexibility and strength." *Journal of Strength and Conditioning Research*, 25, 3391-3398

[8] Mosti MP, Carlsen T, Aas E, Hoff J, Stunes AK, Syversen U. (2014). "Maximal strength training improves bone mineral density and neuromuscular performance in young adult women." *Journal of Strength and Conditioning Research*, 28, 2935

[9] Pedersen, Steen B., et al. "Estrogen controls lipolysis by up-regulating α2A-adrenergic receptors directly in human adipose tissue through the estrogen receptor α. Implications for the female fat distribution." *The Journal of Clinical Endocrinology & Metabolism* 89.4 (2004): 1869-1878.

[10] Stuebe, Alison M., and Janet W. Rich-Edwards. "The reset hypothesis: lactation and maternal metabolism." *American journal of perinatology* 26.01 (2009): 081-088.

[11] Gunderson, Erica P. "The role of lactation in GDM women." *Clinical obstetrics and gynecology* 56.4 (2013): 844.

[12] Ibid.

[13] Wei, Wei, et al. "A clinical study on the short-term effect of berberine in comparison to metformin on the metabolic characteristics of women with polycystic ovary syndrome." *European journal of endocrinology* 166.1 (2012): 99-105.

[14] Ishaque, Sana, et al. "Rhodiola rosea for physical and mental fatigue: a systematic review." *BMC complementary and alternative medicine* 12.1 (2012): 70.

[15] Fothergill, Erin, et al. "Persistent metabolic adaptation 6 years after "The Biggest Loser" competition." *Obesity* 24.8 (2016): 1612-1619.

[16] Treuth et al. "Effects of exercise intensity on 24-h energy expenditure and substrate oxidation." *Medicine and Science in Sports and Exercise*, 28 (1996) 1138-1143.

[17] Tremblay et al. "Impact of exercise intensity on body fatness and skeletal muscle metabolism." *Metabolism.* 43 (1994) 814-818.

[18] Trapp, et al. "The effects of high-intensity intermittent exercise training on fat loss and fasting insulin levels of young women." *International Journal of Obesity*. 2008. 32(4):684-91.

[19] Ibid.

[20] Edwards, et al. "Self-Pacing in interval training: A teleoanticipatory approach." *Psychophysiology*. 2011. 48(1): 136–41.

[21] Ibid.

[22] Williams, et al. "Exercise, affect, and adherence: an integrated model and a case for self-selected exercise." *Journal of Sport and Exercise Psychology*. 2008. 30: 471–496.

[23] Ekkekakis, et al. "Let them roam free? Physiological and psychological evidence for the potential of self-selected exercise intensity in public health." *Sports Medicine*. 2009. 39(10): 857–888.

[24] Duncan, et al. "Exercise motivation: A cross-sectional analysis examining its relationships with frequency, intensity and duration of exercise." *International Journal of Behavioral Nutrition and Physical Activity*. 2010. 7: 7.

[25] Rose, et al. "Exercise experience influences affective and motivational outcomes of prescribed and self-selected intensity exercise." *Scand J Med Sci Sports*. 2012. 22(2): 265–77

[26] Loenneke, et al. "A mechanistic approach to blood flow restriction." *International Journal of Sports Medicine*. 2010. 31(1): 1–4.

[27] la Fleur, Susanne E., et al. "Interaction between corticosterone and insulin in obesity: regulation of lard intake and fat stores." *Endocrinology* 145.5 (2004): 2174-2185.

[28] Pecoraro, Norman, Francisca Gomez, and Mary F. Dallman. "Glucocorticoids dose-dependently remodel energy stores and amplify incentive relativity effects." *Psychoneuroendocrinology* 30.9 (2005): 815-825.

[29] Pecoraro, Norman, et al. "From Malthus to motive: how the HPA axis engineers the phenotype, yoking needs to wants." *Progress in neurobiology* 79.5 (2006): 247-340.

[30] Karjalainen, Eeva, Tytti Sarjala, and Hannu Raitio. "Promoting human health through forests: overview and major challenges." *Environmental health and preventive medicine* 15.1 (2010): 1.

[31] Faraut, Brice, et al. "Napping reverses the salivary interleukin-6 and urinary norepinephrine changes induced by sleep restriction." *The Journal of Clinical Endocrinology & Metabolism* 100.3 (2015): E416-E426.

[32] Ibid.

[33] Ibid.

[34] Young, Deborah Rohm, et al. "Sedentary behavior and cardiovascular morbidity and mortality: a science advisory from the American Heart Association." *Circulation* 134.13 (2016): e262-e279.

[35] Ekelund, Ulf, et al. "Does physical activity attenuate, or even eliminate, the detrimental association of sitting time with mortality? A harmonised meta-analysis of data from more than 1 million men and women." *The Lancet* 388.10051 (2016): 1302-1310.

[36] Henson, J. et al. "Associations of objectively measured sedentary behaviour and physical activity with cardiometabolic health." *Diabetologia*. 2013. 56(5): 1012-20.

[37] Dusca, BD, et al. "Effects of exercise training amount and intensity on peak oxygen consumption in middle-age men and women at risk for cardiovascular disease." *Chest*. 2005. 128(4): 2788-93.

[38] Sampalis, Fotini, et al. "Evaluation of the effects of Neptune Krill Oil™ on the management of premenstrual syndrome and dysmenorrhea." *Alternative medicine review* 8.2 (2003): 171-179.

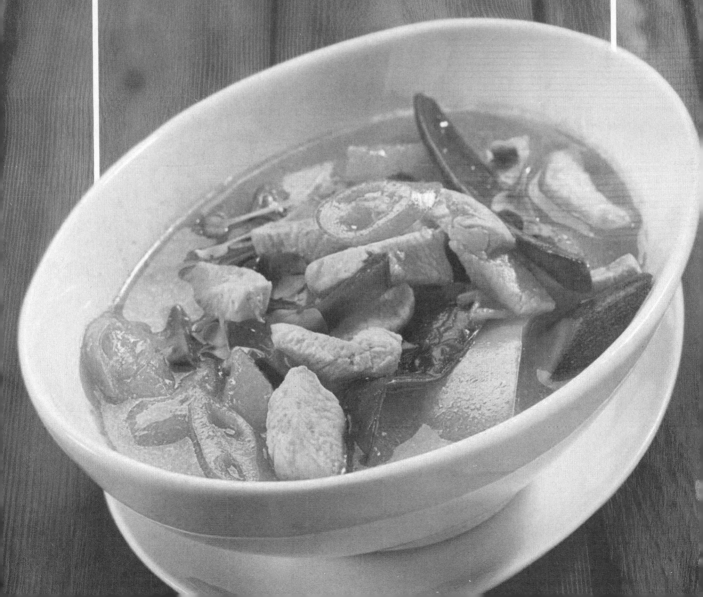

12 WEEK
METABOLIC
MEALS PLAN

TABLE OF CONTENTS

INTRODUCTION

"**Y**ou can't out-train a bad diet." Truer words have seldom been spoken. Even if you exercise day and night, until you get the diet portion of the equation right, it's unlikely that you will achieve your health and fat-loss goals.

In this guide, I have provided you tools and tips to create a meal plan that works for you. You will learn how to "roll your own" meals that will renew your metabolism. You will discover mouthwatering recipes, like Almond Butter Chicken and Savory Steak with Mushrooms, that will please your taste buds as much they do your waistline.

I have added daily meal plans, shopping lists and steps you can take to alter the meal plans according to where you are in your life and in your cycle.

But the number one most important lesson you can take from this guide—from this whole program, actually—is this: There is no one-size-fits-all diet, lifestyle or exercise program. You need to become a metabolic detective and discover what works for you.

To do that, use this book as a guide and follow the AIM protocol outlined in Chapter 7 of *Metabolic Renewal*. Measure your results, pay attention to your SHMEC, and adjust and adapt as needed.

The real key to sustained fat loss and long-term health is to find out what works for you. So don't short-change this process.

Let's get started.

HOW THIS MEAL PLAN WORKS

In the pages that follow you will find information on how to "roll your own" meals, weekly meal plans you can follow if you wish, and dozens of delicious recipes, developed by a professional chef and nutritionist, that are not only mouthwatering, but abide by the highest nutritional standards.

Basically, this book provides a framework for optimizing your diet.

However, there are a few things to keep in mind.

First, the meal plans are built on The 3-2-1 Diet, which is described in detail in *Metabolic Renewal*. You will recall that this diet is structured as follows:

- ✓ 3 meals
- ✓ 2 of those meals have protein and veggies only (a little fruit is allowed)—alternatively, these meals can be shakes
- ✓ 1 of those meals contains a small portion of starch

In the meal plan, you will find that we have included a shake for breakfast on most days of the week. We do it this way because shakes are a quick, convenient, nourishing first meal of the day. People are time-strapped in the morning, and making a 5-minute breakfast shake is often more realistic than cooking a whole breakfast.

However, you don't have to eat this way. You can have a full breakfast and do the shake at lunch. Or you can swap out the shake for any other meal in this plan, or create a "roll your own" meal.

In fact, except in specific cases where I recommend keeping your starch at night (menopausal women, for example), you can pick and choose which meal you eat, swapping out recipes you love with those in the meal plan.

You can also "roll your own" meals some of the time and follow the meal plan other times.

It's all up to you.

You will also discover that there are only three weeks of meal plans in this guide. This is intentional. I have found that most people do not want you to spell out precisely what they are going to eat for the full 12 weeks of the program.

In addition, I want you to get away from the idea that you "must eat this" and "have to avoid that," and focus, instead, on becoming a metabolic detective. I find that three weeks of structured plans provides a good foundation and then people can usually take it from there.

However, if after three weeks, you prefer to follow a structured meal plan, just go back to week one and start over. You can repeat it that way through the entire program, or for as long as you like.

Now the big question you are likely to have is: "How do I adapt this meal plan to fit where I am in my life and with my cycle?"

That's a good question. Let's address each case in detail.

THE NORMALLY MENSTRUATING WOMAN

If you are a normally menstruating woman, you can add one additional meal that includes starch during the first two weeks of your cycle (the follicular phase). In my meal plan, the meals that include starch are dinners. So when creating your additional meal, use my starch suggestions that are provided with dinner meals to help you create your additional meal.

You can add this meal any time it is convenient for you.

Be aware that you do not have to add this meal. It is optional. If you exercise more during this phase of your cycle, you will likely be hungrier and therefore may want to add a little more food to your diet. Thus the addition.

Follow your SHMEC and do what makes sense for you.

During the luteal phase of your cycle, simply drop the additional meal and follow the plan as is.

THE PREGNANT WOMAN

Simply follow the meal plan, and see the sidebar on snacks or add in an additional meal as your hunger dictates. Remember, your body will naturally make you hungrier to help feed your growing baby. Follow that hunger instead of all of the nonsense advice about "eating for two" and I think you will find you are much happier and healthier throughout your pregnancy.

HOW TO CHOOSE THE RIGHT SNACKS

If you are including a snack in your daily routine, your goal is to choose one that provides an ideal mix of fuel for you. A quality snack will carry you to your next meal, keeping your hunger, energy and cravings at bay.

Protein and fiber are often beneficial to achieving this goal. Adding in a small amount of healthy fat can also be helpful for some.

Here are a few snack ideas to try:

- Naked Shake (protein powder plus water or unsweetened non-dairy alternative and ice)

- A low-glycemic fruit, such as an apple or berries

- An apple with a small handful or nuts or 1-2 TB of almond butter

- A hard-boiled egg

- Crudités with hummus

- 2-3 ounces of chicken, turkey or other deli meat with some mixed vegetables

After your baby is born, simply go back to The 3-2-1 Diet as outlined. After 4-8 weeks, you can start cycling the diet as outlined above.

PERIMENOPAUSE, MENOPAUSE, AND POST-MENOPAUSE

There are a few nuances to keep in mind if you are in this stage of life.

First, I particularly like the shakes for women in menopause. Yes, whole foods are probably better, but I find that most of the women I work with in this phase of life are overwhelmed, stressed out and have way too much going on. Cooking a breakfast on top of everything else just adds to that stress load, and we know what stress does for your waistline and your health.

So why add more to a plate that is already full? Just make a shake in the morning instead.

Keep your starch meal in the evening as outlined in these meal plans. I find that it's helpful for sleep, as we discuss in *Metabolic Renewal.*

Do not hesitate to add a snack during your day if you are hungry. This will keep your blood sugar balanced and your stress levels manageable. See the sidebar for more on what snacks to choose.

THE METABOLICALLY CHALLENGED WOMAN

This meal plan as outlined is perfect for you. If you have metabolic challenges, following the meal plan is going to help you reset and rebuild your metabolism.

And one final reminder for everyone: If you follow this program for 7-14 days and either don't see results, or, more importantly, your SHMEC remains out of check, make sure to follow the AIM protocol in Chapter 7 of *Metabolic Renewal.* That process is designed to help you further individualize this program to fit your personal needs.

"ROLL YOUR OWN" SHAKES

We consider the morning shake an essential part of this program for a few reasons:

1. It's easy to make
2. It primes your metabolism
3. It sets you up for a clear, clean pattern of eating for the day

Equally important, the ingredients in it provide the right blend of extremely high-quality protein, fat, fiber and a nice variety of important nutrients, all of which are needed for healthy cells and a smooth-running metabolism.

If you want to "roll your own" shakes, here is what to do.

STEP 1: BEGIN WITH CORE SHAKE INGREDIENTS

✓ **1 Scoop High-Quality Protein Powder.** Your powder should be between 15-25g of protein, less than 6g of carbohydrate, less than 2 grams of sugar and at least 2 grams of dietary fiber. I like whey protein and pea protein.

✓ **1 Tablespoon Chia and/or Flaxseed.** This adds some healthy omega-3s and fiber to your shake.

✓ **⅓ Cup (or Less) of Approved Low- to Moderate-Glycemic Fruit (Optional).** Fruit choices include:

- Berries (blueberries, raspberries, strawberries)
- Cherries
- Pear
- Peach or Nectarine
- Melon
- Orange or Tangerine
- Apple
- Kiwi

✓ **4-8+ Ounces Dairy-Free Liquid.** You may use one liquid alone or a combination of two different liquids (e.g., half water and half unsweetened almond milk). Less liquid may be used if you prefer a thicker consistency shake. Add more liquid if you prefer a thinner consistency shake. Dairy-free liquid choices include:

- Water
- Unsweetened plain almond milk
- Unsweetened plain coconut milk
- Chilled herbal tea

STEP 2: CHOOSE ANY OF THE FOLLOWING SMOOTHIE ADD-IN OPTIONS

The add-ins will provide additional nourishment to your smoothie. Adding nutrients in the form of fiber, fat, and/or starch will help keep you satiated and satisfied for several hours. I recommend that you choose at least 2 items from the list below.

Remember, be a detective. For many people fat is very satiating, and therefore leads to stable SHMEC, less overall calorie intake and better hormonal balance. For others more fiber or more starch will work better. Pay attention to your SHMEC, follow the AIM protocol and discover what works best for you.

Fiber:

- ✓ Additional chia seeds (unsoaked or soaked)[1]
- ✓ 1 tablespoon psyllium husks/powder
- ✓ A handful of leafy greens, like spinach or kale

Healthy Fats:

- ✓ ½-1 ripe avocado
- ✓ ½ cup full-fat canned coconut milk
- ✓ 1 tablespoon unsweetened coconut flakes
- ✓ 1 tablespoon melted coconut oil
- ✓ 1-2 raw pasture eggs
- ✓ ½-1 ounce nuts (e.g., almonds, cashews, walnuts) or 1 tablespoon nut or seed butter (e.g., almond or cashew butter) or 1 tablespoon seeds (e.g., hemp seeds)
- ✓ 1 tablespoon flaxseed oil
- ✓ 1 tablespoon of a delicious fish oil swirl

Starches:

- ✓ ⅓ cup additional fruit, including starchier fruit like banana
- ✓ ½ cup pumpkin (fresh or canned) or other squash
- ✓ ½ cup beets
- ✓ ¼ cup gluten-free oats

You may also consider adding:

- ✓ Additional water or ice depending on how thick or thin you like your shake
- ✓ 1 tablespoon cocoa or cocoa powder for added chocolate flavoring
- ✓ Stevia or xylitol, to taste
- ✓ Lemon or lime rind or juice for extra flavoring
- ✓ 1 tablespoon cinnamon or other herbs
- ✓ 1 scoop of Greens & Reds powder

---

1 To soak chia seeds, mix a few tablespoons into about 6 ounces of water in a small jar and keep in the fridge for about a week. The seeds will expand and gel over time. Mix well to prevent clumping.

STEP 3: BLEND AND ENJOY!

If you're looking for recipes to inspire you, just check out our shake creations. They are delicious and combine protein, fat, fiber and are packed with flavor.

OTHER "ROLL YOUR OWN" BREAKFAST OPTIONS

Of course, shakes aren't the only option for breakfast, so if you want to mix it up or you aren't a big shake person, you can try any smart-carb, medium-protein breakfast. Some options include:

1. Eggs any style, your choice of lean meat, and a small side of fruit.

2. Omelet with your choice of veggies; pile salsa on top and serve with some avocado.

3. Leftovers from the night before. I know this may sound weird, but when you think about it, the traditional American breakfast is just a social convention and not a very healthy one at that. So mix it up. Try a grass-fed bacon burger (no bun) with a side salad. Or go for leftover steak and kale from the night before. Just tune into your body and eat whatever strikes your fancy, as long as it isn't filled with starchy/sugary carbs.

"ROLL YOUR OWN" LUNCHES AND DINNERS

I f you want to "roll your own" lunches and dinners, all you have to do is look at the chart (below) and choose one food from column A and all the items you want from column B.

Then season with, cook with, or include anything from column C that happens to come along with the food listed (meaning, for example, the fat that's found in the fish or in the grass-fed beef) or that makes the food taste better (butter, coconut oil), or is a good accompaniment (avocado).

For your meals that include starch, simply add about ½ cup of any food that is listed in Column D.

It's pure simplicity.

COLUMN A (Protein)	COLUMN B (Vegetables/Fiber)[2]	COLUMN C (Fats and Oils)	COLUMN D (Starch)
Beef	Broccoli	Butter	½ cup sweet potato
Chicken	Cabbage	Ghee	½ cup winter squash (butternut, acorn, etc.)
Eggs	Onions	Coconut oil	½ cup white potato
Turkey	Mushrooms	Avocado oil	½ cup beans
Pasture-raised pork	Spinach	Avocado	½ cup brown rice
Bacon (from pastured pork)	Chard	Palm oil (Malaysian Palm oil is best)	½ cup naturally occurring white rice (jasmine, basmati)
Lamb	Collard greens	Sesame oil (limited)	½ cup quinoa
Salmon	Kale	Flax oil (salad dressing only)	½ cup gluten-free oats
Flounder	Lettuce (romaine, baby spinach, mixed greens, etc.)	Olive oil	½ cup higher glycemic fruit (e.g., banana)
Herring	Bok choy	Macadamia nut oil	
Sardines	Celery	Walnut oil (salad dressing only)	
Sole	Zucchini	Nuts (limit to about 1 ounce per day)	
Tuna	Brussels sprouts		
Trout	Scallions		
Cod	Snow peas / snap peas		
Halibut	Tomatoes		
Sashimi	Artichokes		
Shrimp	Pumpkin		
Scallops	Spaghetti squash		
Clams	Cauliflower		
Crabmeat	Carrots (limit 2 per day)		
Mussels	Green beans		
Oysters			
Lobster			
Veal			
Venison			
Duck			
Ostrich			
Buffalo			
Bison			

2 A note about column B—the vegetables listed here focus on smart-carbs, specifically leafy greens and cruciferous, sulfur-based veggies, all of which are excellent for detoxification. I encourage you to make these your main vegetables sources during the program.

Obviously, the options here are endless, but here are a few sample lunches and dinners you may choose based on the list above:

1. Poached salmon with ½ avocado, ½ plate of mixed vegetables that have been cooked in 1-2 tablespoons coconut oil
2. Grass-fed steak, mashed cauliflower with grass-fed butter and seasonings, a side of sautéed kale
3. Dark meat turkey burger, ½ cup asparagus, ½ cup sautéed onions and peppers, a pat of butter on vegetables
4. Grilled chicken breasts with a large sautéed kale salad, and ½ of a sweet potato with drizzled coconut oil
5. Large 3-egg omelet (including 1-3 yolks depending on SHMEC) loaded with veggies of your choice and a side of ½ cup of hash browns sautéed with onions and garlic

That's all there is to "rolling your own" meals for the *Metabolic Renewal* program.

Now, if you want to make all of this extremely easy on yourself, the meal plans and recipes on the pages that follow will make optimizing your nutrition even easier. These meals were created by a professional recipe developer to adhere to our stringent nutritional guidelines, and are spectacularly delicious and incredibly filling.

Enjoy!

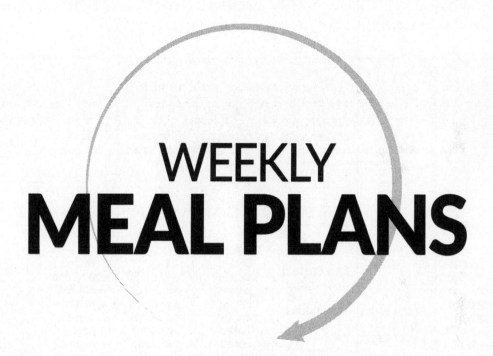

WEEKLY MEAL PLANS

A NOTE ON SERVING SIZES IN THE RECIPES

In the recipes below, you will find the yield—the number of servings the recipe produces—listed at the top of the page. Most of the recipes are designed to feed a family of four. If you are doing the program on your own, simply cut the recipe and shopping list in half. You can also store leftovers in the fridge, and eat them the next day, or freeze them for longer-term storage.

MEAL PLANS: WEEK 1

You will find the recipes that correspond to this meal plan below.

	Monday	Tuesday	Wednesday	Thursday	Friday	Saturday	Sunday
Breakfast	Raspberry Lime Shake	Carrot Cake Shake	"Roll Your Own" Shake	Peachy Nutmeg Shake	Mocha Fudge Shake	Greens and Leeks Omelet	"Roll Your Own" Shake
Lunch	Tuna Artichoke Wraps	Easy Meat Roll-Up	10-Minute Chicken Soup with side salad	Chopped Salad	"Roll Your Own" Salad	Salad Nicoise	Chicken Mesclun Salad
Dinner	Chicken Cacciatore with ½ of a medium sweet potato and a side of Lemony Asparagus	Paleo Fajitas with ½ cup of black beans	Easy Roasted Herb Chicken with ½ cup of butternut squash and a side of Sesame Spinach	Slow-Cooker Coconut Salmon with ½ of medium baked potato and a side of Garlic Broccoli	Turkey Chili with ½ cup brown rice and a small "Roll Your Own' side salad	Grilled Lamb Chops with ½ of a medium sweet potato and a side of Gingered Bok Choy	Slow-Cooker Pork Loin with Mustard and Rosemary with ½ cup of butternut squash and a side of Dijon Asparagus

MEAL PLANS: WEEK 2

You will find the recipes that correspond to this meal plan below.

	Monday	Tuesday	Wednesday	Thursday	Friday	Saturday	Sunday
Breakfast	Black Forest Cherry Cake Shake	Coconut Chai Shake	Roll Your Own Shake	Salted Dark Chocolate Shake	Choco-Nutter Shake	Breakfast Stack	Raspberry Lime Shake
Lunch	California Salad	Shrimp Wraps with side salad	Southwestern Steak Salad	Salmon Burger over mixed green salad	Roll Your Own Salad	Tahini Chicken Salad	Mediterranean Lunch Wrap with side salad
Dinner	Rainbow Stuffed Peppers with ½ cup of black beans and a side of Sesame Spinach	Savory Steak with Mushrooms with ½ of a medium sweet potato and a side of Grilled Peppers and Onions	Grilled Chicken Breasts in Tomato Sauce with ½ a cup of acorn squash and a side of Zucchini and Spinach with Brown Butter	Mini Meatball Minestrone Soup with ½ cup of brown rice and a small "Roll Your Own" side salad	Quick Indian Turkey Burger Salad with ½ cup of quinoa	Slow Cooker Shrimp Diavolo with ½ of a medium baked potato and a side of Broccoli Almondine	Herbed Lamb Kebabs with Grilled Zucchini, ½ of a medium sweet potato and a side of Garlic Broccoli

MEAL PLANS: WEEK 3

You will find the recipes that correspond to this meal plan below.

METABOLIC MEALS PLAN

	Monday	Tuesday	Wednesday	Thursday	Friday	Saturday	Sunday
Breakfast	Mint Chocolate Crunch Shake	Blueberry Eye Opener Shake	Roll Your Own Shake	Chocolate Raspberry Shake	Peachy Nutmeg Shake	Poached Eggs and Turkey Sausage	Roll Your Own Shake
Lunch	Roast Beef Wraps	Pesto Chicken Salad	Italian Sweet Veggie Scramble	Steak Salad	Roll Your Own Salad	Coconut Herbed Frittata	Salmon Wraps
Dinner	Chicken Marsala with ½ a cup of a medium sweet potato and a side of Gingered Bok Choy	Flavorful Flank Steak with ½ of a medium baked potato and a side of Dijon Asparagus	Sole Filet Over Greens with ½ cup of quinoa	Almond Butter Chicken with ½ of a medium sweet potato and a side of Classic Veggie Stir-Fry	Mouthwatering Meatloaf with ½ of a medium baked potato and a side of Grilled Peppers and Onions	Dijon Salmon Steaks with ½ cup of black beans and a side of Zucchini and Spinach with Brown Butter	Baked Pesto Chicken with ½ of a cup of butternut squash and a side of Garlic Broccoli

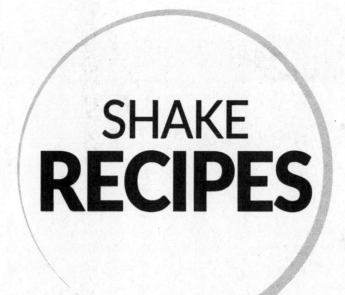

SHAKE
RECIPES

BLACK FOREST CHERRY CAKE SHAKE

Yield: 1 serving

Black forest cake is famous for its luscious dark chocolate and dark cherries. This version has sweet, dark cherries and cocoa nibs that are 100% crushed cocoa bean. If you aren't able to find cocoa nibs, you can swap in unsweetened cocoa powder mixed with a touch of coconut oil.

Ingredients

1 serving protein powder (here's my favorite brand: http://www.metabolicprime.com/protein)
⅓ cup frozen cherries
¼ cup baby spinach
½ cup unsweetened almond milk
4 ice cubes
2 tablespoons chia seeds
1 tablespoon cocoa nibs (or unsweetened cocoa powder)
½ teaspoon almond or vanilla extract

Instructions

Place all ingredients in a blender and process until smooth. Serve immediately.

BLUEBERRY EYE-OPENER SHAKE

Yield: 1 Serving

Wake up your senses with this blueberry and collards delight!

Ingredients

1 serving protein powder
1 cup unsweetened almond milk
½ cup blueberries
1 handful stemmed and chopped young raw collard greens
1 tablespoon chia seed
2 teaspoons stevia (optional)

Instructions

Place all ingredients in the blender and add water to create desired consistency. Process until smooth. Serve immediately.

CARROT CAKE SHAKE

Yield: 1 serving

Carrots, orange and spice blend together for a carrot-cake lover's dream breakfast. Cinnamon is not only a sweet-tasting spice, it packs plenty of antioxidant power and blood-sugar balancing properties.

Ingredients

1 serving protein powder
1 carrot, chopped
¼ cup skin-on apple, chopped
½ cup unsweetened almond milk
4 ice cubes
1 tablespoon walnuts, chopped
1 tablespoon chia seeds
1 tablespoon orange zest
½ teaspoon vanilla extract
½ teaspoon cinnamon
¼ teaspoon nutmeg

Instructions

Place all ingredients in a blender and process until smooth. Serve immediately.

CHOCOLATE RASPBERRY SHAKE

Yield: 1 Serving

Craving chocolate? Adding some raw cocoa or cocoa powder to your shake will help!

Ingredients

1 serving protein powder
1 cup unsweetened almond milk
½ cup frozen raspberries
1 large handful raw baby spinach
1 tablespoon cocoa powder
1 tablespoon chia seed
2 teaspoons stevia (optional)

Instructions

Add all ingredients to blender and blend until very smooth.

CHOCO-NUTTER SHAKE

Yield: 1 Serving

This rich chocolate shake combined with almond butter will delight your senses and help keep your cravings at bay.

Ingredients

1 serving protein powder
1 cup unsweetened almond milk
1 tablespoon almond butter
1 heaping tablespoon raw cacao or cocoa powder
1 tablespoon chia seed
2 teaspoons stevia (optional)

Instructions

Add all ingredients to blender and blend until very smooth.

COCONUT CHAI SHAKE

Yield: 1 serving

Chai tea, fragrant with spices, is popular worldwide because of the warming, comforting taste from cinnamon, nutmeg and cardamom. Not only do these spices tickle your taste buds, they contain vital minerals, like manganese and calcium, plus a wide array of detoxifying compounds.

Ingredients

1 serving protein powder
1 carrot, chopped
½ cup unsweetened coconut milk (from a carton, not canned)
¼ cup shredded unsweetened coconut
4 ice cubes
2 tablespoons chia seeds
½ teaspoon vanilla extract
½ teaspoon cinnamon
¼ teaspoon cardamom or nutmeg

Instructions

Place all ingredients in a blender along with ½ cup water and process until smooth. Serve immediately.

MINT CHOCOLATE CRUNCH SHAKE

Yield: 1 serving

Fresh mint and chocolate make a sweet, refreshing treat. Fatty, rich avocado gives this shake an appealing ice-cream-like texture that you can ramp up with a fun crunch of chopped almonds.

Ingredients

1 serving protein powder
⅓ cup skin-on apple, chopped
⅓ cup avocado, diced
½ cup unsweetened almond milk or coconut milk (from a carton, not canned)
4 ice cubes
2 tablespoons fresh mint leaves, chopped
1 tablespoon unsalted almonds, chopped (optional)
½ teaspoon vanilla extract
1 tablespoon cocoa nibs (or unsweetened cocoa powder)
1 teaspoon stevia (optional)

Instructions

Place all ingredients in a blender along with ½ cup water and process until smooth. Serve immediately.

PEACHY NUTMEG SHAKE

Yield: 1 Serving

Have a peachy breakfast that offers the warming spice of nutmeg.

Ingredients

1 serving protein powder
8 ounces unsweetened almond milk
½ cup frozen peaches
½ teaspoon nutmeg
1 tablespoon chia seeds
2 teaspoons stevia (optional)

Instructions

Add all ingredients to blender and blend until very smooth.

RASPBERRY LIME SHAKE

Yield: 1 Serving

Instead of unsweetened almond milk, this shake uses chilled green tea as its base. The green tea helps kick-start your metabolism. The raspberry and spinach provide your body with additional nourishing nutrients.

Ingredients

1 serving protein powder
8 ounces chilled green tea
½ cup frozen raspberries
Juice and zest from ½ lime
1 tablespoon chia seeds
1 large handful raw baby spinach
2 teaspoons stevia (optional)

Instructions

Place all ingredients in a blender along with ½ cup water and 4 ice cubes. Blend until smooth. Serve immediately.

SALTED DARK CHOCOLATE SHAKE

Yield: 1 serving

If sweet and salty is your thing, this shake has your name on it! Chia adds thickness and crunch. Dark chocolate, a powerful superfood, is being studied as a high-powered nutrient for memory support.

Ingredients

1 serving protein powder
½ cup kale, chopped
½ cup unsweetened almond or coconut milk (from carton, not canned)
4 ice cubes
1 tablespoon cocoa powder
2 tablespoons chia seeds
½ teaspoon vanilla extract
½ teaspoon cinnamon
⅛ teaspoon sea salt
2 tablespoons cocoa nibs
1 teaspoon stevia (optional)

Instructions

Place all ingredients in a blender except cocoa nibs. Process until smooth. Stir in cocoa nibs. Serve immediately.

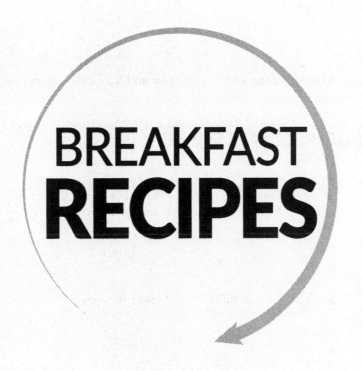

BREAKFAST RECIPES

BREAKFAST STACK

Yield: 1 serving

Get your omega-3s first thing in the morning with a serving of wild salmon for breakfast. This stack is packed with nutrition that will fuel you until lunchtime.

Ingredients

2 teaspoons olive oil
2-3 eggs
Salt and freshly ground pepper to taste
3 ounces smoked wild salmon
2 prepared roasted red pepper halves
¼ avocado, thinly sliced
4 thin red onion rings

Instructions

Heat the olive oil in a large skillet over medium heat and crack the eggs carefully into the pan. Season the eggs lightly with salt and pepper. Cook to desired doneness, flipping once.

Transfer the cooked eggs onto a plate and layer with smoked wild salmon, red pepper, avocado slices and onion rings.

GREENS AND LEEKS OMELET

Yield: 1 Serving

Get your morning dose of greens in this easy omelet that's loaded with plenty of flavor and substance.

Ingredients

2 teaspoons olive oil
¼ cup collard greens, kale and spinach, stemmed and finely chopped
¼ cup finely chopped leek
1 tablespoon water
½ teaspoon each salt and freshly ground pepper
2-3 eggs

Instructions

Heat the olive oil in a 12-inch non-stick skillet over medium heat. Add the greens, leeks and 1 tablespoon water. Cover for 2 minutes. Cook, stirring occasionally, until the vegetables are tender, 2-4 minutes.

While the veggies are cooking, combine the eggs, salt, pepper and water in a small bowl and whisk until lightly beaten. When the vegetables are tender, increase the heat to medium-high for 1 minute. Pour the eggs evenly over the veggies and allow to sit undisturbed, for 1 minute.

Working gently, lift one half of the omelet and flip it over the other half. Cook for about 30 seconds and flip once to cook to desired doneness.

POACHED EGGS AND TURKEY SAUSAGE

Yield: 2 servings

For an extra protein punch, pair your eggs with some gluten-free turkey sausage. If you purchase the precooked variety, you can gently heat and have this substantial breakfast served in a matter of minutes.

Ingredients

2 teaspoons coconut oil
½ pound Italian gluten-free turkey sausage, thinly sliced
1 pint cherry or grape tomatoes, halved
2 eggs

Instructions

Place a small covered saucepan half full of water over medium-high heat to boil. Heat the coconut oil in a large skillet over medium heat and add the sausage. Cook for about 5 minutes and add the tomatoes, cooking for an additional 3-4 minutes or until sausage is cooked through and tomatoes are hot and soft.

When the water comes to a simmer, remove the lid and carefully crack the eggs into a small bowl without breaking the yolks. Slowly and carefully slide them out of the bowl and into the simmering water, up against the side of the pan, if possible. Simmer the eggs for 3-5 minutes to desired doneness and carefully remove them with a slotted spoon. Serve the eggs over the sausage and tomatoes.

LUNCH
RECIPES

CALIFORNIA SALAD

Yield: 4 Servings

Sunny California skies and balmy weather mean fresh produce year 'round, like the tomatoes and avocado that you'll enjoy in this out-of-the-ordinary salad. Seasoned chicken and smoky bacon add plenty of savory flavor and help you feel full longer.

Ingredients

2 skinless, boneless chicken breasts
½ teaspoon chili powder, mild or hot
½ teaspoon garlic powder
¼ teaspoon salt
¼ teaspoon freshly ground black pepper
1 tablespoon coconut oil
6 cups mixed greens
2 slices bacon, chopped
2 tablespoons balsamic vinegar
2 garlic cloves
2 cups cherry tomatoes, halved
1 avocados, sliced

Instructions

Sprinkle the chicken with chili powder, garlic powder, salt and pepper. Heat a large skillet over high heat and add the coconut oil. Add the chicken and reduce the heat to medium. Cook 7-8 minutes, turning once or twice until the chicken is cooked through and no longer pink in the center. Transfer the chicken to a cutting board and rest 5 minutes before slicing. In the same skillet, place the bacon. Warm the skillet over medium heat and cook 4-5 minutes, stirring often until the bacon is crisp. Transfer the bacon to the plate. Pour off half the bacon fat, then add the balsamic vinegar and garlic. Stir well and set aside.

Spread the greens out on a platter. Sprinkle with the bacon, tomatoes, avocado and the balsamic mixture in the skillet. Add the chicken, divide and serve.

Short on time? Use leftover cooked chicken to create this salad in minutes.

CHICKEN MESCLUN SALAD

Yield: 4 servings

This basic salad gets dressed up with delicious red pepper, pine nuts and vinegar flavoring. Mesclun greens originated from France but can be found at your local grocer. Or, if you prefer, try a mix of other greens like arugula, romaine, kale or spinach.

Ingredients

Dressing
3 prepared roasted red peppers, drained, and divided (or make your own*)
2 tablespoons pine nuts
1 small shallot, peeled and quartered
2 tablespoons red wine vinegar
½ teaspoon Dijon mustard
¼ teaspoon each salt and freshly ground pepper
1 tablespoons olive oil

Salad
6 cups mesclun greens
1 pint grape tomatoes
1 cup chopped cucumber, peeled and seeded
⅔ cup shredded carrots
2 cups cubed chicken, cooked
1 ripe avocados, sliced

Instructions

Combine 1 of the roasted red peppers with all the dressing ingredients and three tablespoons of water in a food processor. Process until mostly smooth. Set aside.

Dice the remaining 2 roasted red peppers. In a large salad bowl, combine the peppers, lettuce, tomatoes, cucumber, carrots, chicken and avocado. Toss gently to combine. Dress to taste. Serve immediately.

*To roast fresh bell peppers, preheat broiler, slice peppers in half lengthwise, remove stems and veins and clap together to remove seeds. Place face down on a broiler sheet and broil for 10-15 minutes or until skin is charred. Remove peppers, place in a bowl, and seal tightly with plastic wrap for 10 minutes. Remove wrap, slip off and discard charred skins.

CHOPPED SALAD

Yield: 4 servings

Chopped salad is quite popular at many take-out salad spots. This do-it-yourself version can be prepped ahead of time by chopping up some of the ingredients and storing them in the fridge until you're ready to eat.

Ingredients

6 cups romaine lettuce, chopped
2 cups baby spinach
12 ounces cooked turkey breast, chopped
2 hard-boiled eggs, peeled and chopped
1 medium avocado, chopped
½ medium cucumber, peeled and chopped
1 slice cooked bacon, chopped
1 tablespoon red onion, finely chopped
4 tablespoons extra-virgin olive oil
½ teaspoon Dijon mustard
2 tablespoons apple cider vinegar
A pinch of salt and freshly ground black pepper

Instructions

In a large salad bowl, add the chopped lettuce, baby spinach, turkey breast, avocado, cucumber, bacon and onion.

In a small bowl, combine the olive oil, Dijon mustard, cider vinegar, salt and pepper until lightly emulsified. Drizzle dressing over the salad, and toss. Serve immediately.

COCONUT HERBED FRITTATA

Yield: 4 servings

A coconut-herbal infusion makes this frittata a warming and satisfying meal. You'll just need 15-20 minutes to create this scrumptious lunch.

Ingredients

2 tablespoons coconut oil
6 eggs, separated into whites and yolks
½ teaspoon salt
¼ teaspoon freshly ground pepper
¼ cup fresh cilantro, chopped
¼ cup fresh basil, chopped

Instructions

Preheat oven to 350°F. Place oil in a 12-inch cast iron skillet (or other oven-safe pan) and place in the oven to melt. Remove the pan as soon as the oil is melted and swirl to coat the bottom of the pan. Pour the remaining oil into a medium bowl to cool.

Transfer the egg whites to a mixer bowl and beat until stiff peaks form. Set aside. Add the egg yolks, salt and pepper to the cooled oil and whisk until well combined. Fold the egg yolks, cilantro and basil gently into the egg whites and pour into the skillet. Bake for 15 minutes or until cooked through and remove carefully with a spatula. Slice and serve.

EASY MEAT ROLL-UP

Yield: 2 Servings

Disguise your vegetables in these protein roll-ups. They are an easy on-the-go lunch that can be prepared ahead of time and sealed closed with a toothpick. If you need a little more protein or fat to keep you full longer, add some extra deli meat and/or some slices of avocado.

Ingredients

Roll-up
1 cup broccoli slaw (or other shredded veggies of choices)
6 ounces sliced gluten-free deli meat of your choice (roast beef, chicken, turkey, etc.)
1 tomato, seeded and chopped
3 tablespoons homemade mayonnaise

Mayonnaise
1 whole egg
½ teaspoon of Dijon mustard or 1 teaspoon dry mustard powder
2 tablespoons lemon juice
¼ teaspoon salt
1 cup light olive oil

Instructions

Prepare the mayonnaise. Add all mayonnaise ingredients to a wide mouth Mason jar. Let the oil rise to the top. Place immersion blender at the very bottom of the jar and blend. As the mayo emulsifies, slowly tilt the immersion blender to allow the remaining oil to blend. Store any unused portion refrigerated, in an airtight container and use within two weeks.
In medium bowl, combine the shredded veggies, tomato and mayonnaise and mix gently to evenly coat. Spread the filling onto deli meat and roll up tightly to enclose the filling.

ITALIAN SWEET VEGGIE SCRAMBLE

Yield: 1 Serving

The flavors of Italy can be enjoyed in this easy-to-prepare scrambled egg dish. Add some avocado or olives if you need a healthy fat boost.

Ingredients

2 teaspoons coconut oil
3 tablespoons minced sweet onion
½ seeded and diced red or orange bell pepper
4 grape tomatoes, quartered
2 eggs
½ teaspoon dried basil
½ teaspoon each salt and freshly ground pepper

Instructions

Heat the coconut oil in a skillet over medium heat. Add the onions and peppers and cover for 2 minutes. Remove cover, add the tomatoes and cook, stirring occasionally, until all the veggies have softened.

While the vegetables are cooking, combine the eggs, basil, salt, and pepper in a small bowl and whisk until lightly beaten.

When the veggies reach desired tenderness, pour the egg mixture over the vegetables. Using a spatula to turn the eggs and veggies occasionally, cook for a few minutes to desired doneness.

MEDITERRANEAN LUNCH WRAP

Yield: 1 Serving

Add some Mediterranean flair to your egg wrap with fresh tomatoes, Kalamata olives and basil. Eggs are an easy and very quick lunch option.

Ingredients

2 eggs
1 cooked turkey or chicken sausage
Pinch of salt and freshly ground pepper
1 tablespoon olive oil

⅓ cup diced tomatoes
2 tablespoons Kalamata olives, pitted and finely diced
Fresh basil

Instructions

In a small bowl, whisk eggs, salt and pepper together until well mixed. Heat olive oil in a large nonstick skillet over medium heat. When pan is well heated, pour in the eggs and swirl the contents until they coat the entire bottom surface of the pan very thinly.

When the egg sets, loosen the bottom with a large spatula and slide it carefully onto a larger flat platter in one large piece. Cover the egg evenly with room temperature or hot sausage, tomatoes, olives and basil, and gently roll up away from you like a cigar. Slice in half with a sharp knife and serve immediately.

PESTO CHICKEN SALAD

Yield: 4 Servings

Delight your senses by combining basil, garlic, olive oil and pine nuts to create this easy pesto sauce that turns your typical chicken salad into a gourmet delight.

Ingredients

12-ounce bag broccoli slaw mix
2 cups diced cooked white chicken
1 cup basil or baby arugula
1 garlic clove

¼ cup pine nuts
3-4 tablespoons olive oil
Salt and pepper to taste
Mixed greens

Instructions

Prepare a vegan pesto by combining the basil (or arugula), garlic, pine nuts, olive oil, salt and pepper in a food processor. Process until chopped and well blended, scraping the sides as necessary. Combine the slaw mix, chicken and pesto in a large bowl and mix well to coat. Pile the pesto mix onto mixed greens or on lettuce leaves to wrap.

ROAST BEEF WRAPS

Yield: 2 Servings

Keep deli roast beef on hand for this simple lunchtime meal that can be created in less than 5 minutes. If you aren't a fan of roast beef, use another deli meat such as turkey or chicken.

Ingredients

2 packed cups baby spinach
¾ cup carrots
2 teaspoons finely minced fresh ginger or fresh-squeezed lemon juice
12 thin slices high-quality gluten-free deli roast beef
1 avocado, peeled, and mashed into a paste

Instructions

Combine the spinach and carrots in a food processor and pulse until finely chopped, but not pureed, scraping down the sides as necessary. Stir in ginger or lemon juice.

Double up the roast beef slices and lay out 6 roast beef "wraps." Spread equal amounts of the avocado onto each wrap. Spoon out equal portions of the spinach carrot mixture over the avocado and tightly roll the beef wraps.

Serve immediately.

"ROLL YOUR OWN" SALAD

Yield: 4 Servings

Taking a trip to the salad bar is fun because it means plenty of options! So, set up a salad bar at home using the following ingredients, or substitute with your own favorites. Prep ingredients and store in partitioned storage containers in your fridge so your salad bar is ready any time you open your fridge.

Ingredients

Suggested Base
4 cups salad greens
4 cups romaine lettuce, chopped
1 cup green beans, steamed
1 cup broccoli florets, raw
1 cup artichokes, quartered

Suggested Toppings
Protein of your choice (cooked chicken, turkey, lean steak, etc.)
½ cup pitted black or green olives
1 avocado
Bacon, crumbled
½ ounce nuts or seeds (e.g., walnuts, almonds, macadamia nuts, sunflower seeds)
1 cup bean sprouts
1 cup homemade pickles (optional)

Suggested Dressings
Lime Dressing
1 lime, zested and juiced (about 2 tablespoons)
1 tablespoon coconut oil, melted
1 teaspoon Dijon mustard
Combine ingredients and whisk well. This dressing must be stored at room temperature so that the coconut oil does not solidify.

Balsamic Dressing
¼ cup coconut oil
¼ cup balsamic vinegar
¼ teaspoon salt
¼ teaspoon freshly ground pepper
Combine ingredients and whisk well. This dressing must be stored at room temperature so that the coconut oil does not solidify.

Basil Vinaigrette Dressing
⅓ cup chicken broth, low-sodium
1 tablespoon fresh basil, chopped
1 tablespoon extra-virgin olive oil
1 tablespoon fresh lemon juice
1 tablespoon apple cider vinegar
1 garlic clove, minced

1 teaspoon Dijon mustard
Freshly ground pepper, to taste
Using a blender, combine all ingredients and process until smooth.

Parsley Basil Dressing
1 packed cup flat leaf parsley, lower stems removed (about 1 small bunch)
½ cup loosely packed fresh basil leaves
1 clove garlic, crushed
2 tablespoons red wine vinegar
Salt and freshly ground pepper, to taste
¼ cup extra-virgin olive oil
Combine everything but the olive oil in a food processor. Pulse together, then drizzle the oil in a thin stream, scraping down the sides frequently, until smooth, creamy and bright green.

Herb Dressing
3 tablespoons extra virgin olive oil
2 tablespoons flaxseed oil (optional)
Juice of 1 lemon
2 teaspoons red wine vinegar
2 cloves garlic, minced
1 teaspoon dried oregano
½ teaspoon dried basil
Salt and freshly ground pepper, to taste
Combine ingredients and whisk well.

Instructions

Mix and match from the base and toppings category to make the salad of your choice! Serve with one of the recommended dressings.

Note: Store-bought pickles can be high in sodium and contain sugar. For easy homemade pickles, place ½ cup vinegar in a saucepan with ½ teaspoon salt and a handful of fresh dill. Bring to a boil, and add 4 peeled cucumbers cut into chunks. Turn the heat off and cover. Rest for 30 minutes then chill. Store in the fridge for two or more weeks.

SALAD NICOISE

Yield: 4 Servings

This recipe is a twist on a classic French salad. Use your creativity to dress it up with other fresh vegetables, such as steamed cauliflower or broccoli, or keep it simple and traditional with the tomatoes and green beans.

Ingredients

2 5-ounce cans chunk light tuna packed in extra virgin olive oil, well drained
1 15-ounce jar artichoke hearts, well drained and coarsely chopped
2 eggs, hard-boiled and quartered
1½ tablespoon capers, drained, or to taste
6 cups romaine lettuce, chopped
½ cup black olives, pitted and drained
1 pint cherry tomatoes
¼ red onion, very thinly sliced
2 cups cut fresh or frozen green beans, prepared according to package directions
¼ teaspoon salt
¼ teaspoon freshly ground pepper

Herb Dressing
3 tablespoons extra-virgin olive oil
2 tablespoons flaxseed oil (optional)
Juice of 1 lemon
2 teaspoons red wine vinegar
2 cloves garlic, minced
1 teaspoon dried oregano
½ teaspoon dried basil
Salt and freshly ground pepper, to taste

Instructions

In a medium bowl, combine the tuna, artichoke hearts and capers, and fold in a portion of the herb dressing to coat.

In a large salad bowl, make a bed of lettuce. Add the olives, tomatoes, onions, and green beans, and spoon tuna evenly over the top. Add the quartered hard-boiled eggs.

For the dressing, combine all ingredients and whisk well. Pour desired amount of dressing evenly over the salad.

SALMON BURGER

Yield: 4 Servings

There's very little preparation time needed for these healthy burgers that are loaded in omega-3s. Pair with a side of vegetables to complete this heart and brain healthy meal.

Ingredients

1 egg
2 7.5-ounce cans wild salmon
⅓ cup almond flour
1 tablespoon lemon zest
1 tablespoon fresh dill, finely chopped
1 tablespoon capers, rinsed and drained
1 teaspoon Dijon mustard
Coconut oil to lightly coat pan
1 lemon, quartered
¼ cup onions, chopped
1 ripe avocado, sliced

Instructions

In a medium bowl, lightly beat the egg. Add the salmon, almond flour, lemon zest, dill, capers, mustard and onions. Mix well to thoroughly combine, and shape firmly into 4 patties.

Lightly coat large skillet with coconut oil and place over medium heat. Cook 4-5 minutes per side or until lightly browned on each side and cooked through. Squeeze ¼ lemon over each patty. Add avocado sliced on top of burgers.

SALMON WRAPS

Yield: 1 Serving

Use precooked salmon for this recipe or, to keep your lunch even simpler, purchase canned wild salmon and drain any excess juices. There will be leftover dressing so use it again on another salad or in a wrap of your choice!

Ingredients

½ cup boneless, skinless cooked salmon
2 tablespoons cucumber, finely diced
2 tablespoons celery, finely diced
2 teaspoons red onion, minced
Romaine leaves
1 tablespoon chopped tomato
2-4 tablespoons Basil Vinaigrette Dressing

Basil Vinaigrette Dressing
⅓ cup chicken broth, low-sodium
1 tablespoon fresh basil, chopped
1 tablespoon extra-virgin olive oil
1 tablespoon fresh lemon juice
1 tablespoon apple cider vinegar
1 garlic clove, minced
1 teaspoon Dijon mustard
Freshly ground pepper, to taste

Instructions

For the dressing: combine all ingredients in a blender.

For the salad: In a small bowl, combine the salmon, cucumber, celery, onion and vinaigrette. Mix well. Lay the mixture out on the romaine leaves and top with tomato. Roll up and serve. Store leftover dressing for future use.

SHRIMP WRAPS

Yield: 4 Servings

Get your seafood fix at lunch with these delicate Asian-inspired wraps. Add a side of veggies and you can season those with the lime, too!

Ingredients

8 large lettuce leaves
2 tablespoons sesame oil
2 tablespoons fresh ginger, minced
24 ounces medium shrimp, shelled and deveined
¼ teaspoon cayenne pepper
1 tablespoon tamari (gluten-free)
1 lime, halved

Instructions

Lay out 4 plates with 2 lettuce leaves each and set aside. Heat the sesame oil over medium in a large skillet.

Add the ginger and sauté 1 minute. Add the shrimp and season with cayenne pepper. Cook, stirring frequently, for 2 minutes. Add the tamari, toss lightly, and cook for another minute or until shrimp just turns pink. Divide shrimp evenly among the lettuce wraps. Squeeze lime on top. Serve immediately.

SOUTHWESTERN STEAK SALAD

Yield: 4 Servings

This savory steak salad with creamy lime dressing that clings to the leaves will soon be a regular on your lunch or dinner plate. Leftover meat for additional salads can be stored for up to 3 days. You can also make this salad quickly by using leftover prepared steak.

Ingredients

Steak

1½ pound flank steak
2 garlic cloves, minced
1 teaspoon coconut oil
½ teaspoon salt
1 teaspoon chili powder
½ teaspoon ground cumin

Salad

8 ounces romaine lettuce, chopped
1 cup thinly sliced raw red bell pepper or grilled peppers and onions (see Vegetable Sides)
¼ cup cilantro leaves
2 tablespoons pickled jalapeños, chopped (optional)

Zesty Lime Dressing

1 lime, zested and juiced (about 2 tablespoons)
1 tablespoon coconut oil
1 teaspoon Dijon mustard

Instructions

Heat a large skillet or grill over medium heat. Rub the steak with the garlic cloves, coconut oil, salt, chili powder, and cumin. Transfer the steak to the skillet or grill and cook 8-10 minutes (or less if a thinner cut of meat), turning occasionally until the meat is pink in the center but not translucent. Rest 5 minutes on a cutting board and thinly slice against the grain.

For the dressing, Place the lime zest and juice in a small bowl. Add the coconut oil and mustard. Whisk well.

Add the romaine, grilled peppers or red bell pepper, cilantro and pickled jalapeños, if using. Pour the dressing over vegetables. Top with the flank steak. Serve immediately.

STEAK SALAD

Yield: 4 Servings

The parsley-basil sauce will bring enjoyment to your senses and perfectly complement the flank steak.

Ingredients

1 packed cup fresh parsley, lower stems removed (about 1 small bunch)
½ cup loosely packed fresh basil leaves
1 clove garlic, crushed
2 tablespoons red wine vinegar
¼ teaspoon each salt and freshly ground pepper, or to taste
¼ cup olive oil
1 24-ounce flank steak
6 cups mesclun salad greens
½ small red onion, thinly sliced

Instructions

Preheat the grill to medium-high.

Combine the parsley, basil, garlic, vinegar, salt and pepper in a food processor. Start to process and drizzle the oil in a thin stream, scraping down the sides frequently until the mixture is smooth, creamy and bright green. Set aside.

Season the flank steak lightly with salt and pepper, and grill for about 7 minutes per side for medium rare. Let rest for at least 5 minutes, and slice thinly across the grain. Make 4 beds of the lettuce greens; top each with equal portions of the onion and steak, and dress to taste with the parsley-basil sauce or other dressing of choice.

TAHINI CHICKEN SALAD

Yield: 4 Servings

Tahini is a rich paste that's made from ground sesame seeds and is sometimes called sesame paste or sesame butter. The paste goes very well with versatile meat, such as chicken breast.

Ingredients

1 clove garlic, crushed
¼ cup tahini
Juice and zest of ½ lemon
1 tablespoon apple cider vinegar
1 teaspoon tamari (gluten-free)
2 cooked boneless, skinless chicken breasts, diced or shredded
1½ cups raw or blanched green veggies (e.g., 1-inch green beans, broccoli florets, chopped sugar snap peas, diced bell pepper, etc.)
1 cup grape tomatoes
¼ cup almonds, sliced
¼ cup pitted black olives
8-12 large lettuce leaves

Instructions

Combine tahini, lemon juice and zest, cider vinegar, tamari and 2 tablespoons of water in a food processor. Process until smooth, scraping down the sides as necessary. If dressing is too thick or sticky, add more water a tablespoon at a time. Transfer dressing to a medium bowl, add chicken, green veggies, tomatoes, almonds and olives, and toss gently to coat well. Serve over lettuce leaves.

10-MINUTE CHICKEN SOUP

Yield: 4 Servings

Nothing is more soothing than a bowl of chicken soup and this quick version can be made in less than 10 minutes.

Ingredients

2 tablespoons coconut oil
1 onion, chopped
2 garlic cloves, minced
1 tablespoon ginger, minced
4 cups chicken broth, low-sodium
2 cups broccoli florets
2 cups cauliflower florets
2 cups cooked white chicken, shredded or diced
¼ cup fresh basil leaves, sliced

Instructions

Heat a large stockpot over medium heat. Add the coconut oil along with the onions, garlic and minced ginger. Cook 1-2 minutes, stirring often, until the onions soften. Add the chicken broth, broccoli and cauliflower. Cook until the broccoli and cauliflower are tender. Stir in the chicken and fresh basil. Simmer until pieces of chicken are hot.

TUNA ARTICHOKE WRAPS

Yield: 2-3 Servings

Instead of a tuna salad, try these lettuce wraps, which provide plenty of healthy fats from the green olives, olive oil and avocado slices. The artichokes are an antioxidant-rich food and a great source of dietary fiber, folate and vitamins C and K.

Ingredients

1 15-ounce jar artichoke hearts in water, drained
½ cup pitted green olives
2 5-ounce cans chunk light tuna in extra-virgin olive oil, well drained
2 teaspoons capers, rinsed to remove excess salt
2 teaspoons extra-virgin olive oil
Juice and zest of ½ small lemon
Salt, to taste
½ avocado, sliced
Romaine leaves for wraps

Instructions

Combine the artichoke hearts and olives in a food processor and pulse until well chopped and mixed, but retaining some chunkiness. Transfer contents to a medium bowl and stir in the tuna, capers, olive oil, lemon juice and zest and salt until well mixed. Adjust seasonings, if necessary. Spoon small amounts into lettuce and top with slices of avocado. Wrap and serve.

DINNER
RECIPES

ALMOND BUTTER CHICKEN

Yield: 4 Servings

Use your leftover almond butter from morning shakes to create this simple chicken dish. The nutty, rich flavoring of the almond butter compliments the chicken breasts. This recipe will soon become a family standby.

Ingredients

3 tablespoons olive oil, divided
3 tablespoons lemon juice, divided
½ teaspoon ground cumin
¼ teaspoon salt
4 large boneless, skinless chicken breasts
1 medium onion
¼ teaspoon garlic powder
⅓ cup almond butter

Instructions

In a glass storage container, combine 2 tablespoons each of olive oil, lemon juice, cumin and salt. Add the chicken and marinate 10-60 minutes.

Preheat oven broiler. Place chicken breasts on broiler sheet and broil for about 6-7 minutes per side or until cooked through but still juicy.

While the chicken is cooking, heat the remaining tablespoon of olive oil in a skillet over medium heat. Add the onion and sauté for about 6 minutes or until translucent. Add ½ cup water, the garlic powder and remaining tablespoon of lemon juice. Bring the mixture to a boil and remove from heat. Whisk in the almond butter until melted and incorporated.

Pour the sauce over the chicken and serve warm.

BAKED PESTO CHICKEN

Yield: 4 Servings

Let your senses take you to Italy with this pesto chicken recipe that takes only 30 minutes to cook. It goes very well with a side of vegetables and a side salad.

Ingredients

1¼ pounds chicken breasts
1 cup basil or baby arugula
1 garlic clove, crushed
¼ cup pine nuts, toasted
4 tablespoons olive oil
Salt and freshly ground pepper to taste

Instructions

Preheat the oven to 350 degrees.

Make pesto by combining the basil or arugula, garlic, pine nuts, olive oil, salt and pepper in a food processor. Process until chopped and well blended, scraping down sides as necessary.

Arrange the chicken breasts in a single layer 11x7-inch baking pan. Spoon pesto evenly over the top and distribute over the chicken with a knife. Bake for 30-35 minutes until cooked through and juicy.

CHICKEN CACCIATORE

Yield: 4 Servings

Chicken cacciatore means "chicken hunter-style." It gets its delicious sauce from the foraged wild mushrooms hunters would find in the forest. You won't have to hunt for long as this tasty dish takes under 20 minutes to make. This recipe works well with any type of store-bought mushrooms.

Ingredients

¾ pound chicken breasts (about 4 chicken breasts)
1 teaspoon dried oregano
1 teaspoon chopped fresh or dried rosemary
¼ teaspoon freshly ground black pepper
¼ teaspoon salt
3 tablespoons butter, preferably grass-fed
1 5-ounce package mushrooms, thinly sliced
½ red bell pepper, thinly sliced
¼ cup thinly sliced onion
1 teaspoon chili powder
1 teaspoon garlic powder
4 cups baby spinach
½ lemon, zested and juiced

Instructions

Preheat oven or toaster oven to 400°F. Cover a baking sheet with aluminum foil. Sprinkle the chicken with oregano, rosemary, black pepper, and salt. Place the seasoned chicken skin side up on the foil. Bake 30 to 35 minutes until no longer pink at the bone.

While the chicken cooks, prepare the sauce. Warm the butter in a large skillet over medium heat and add the mushrooms, bell pepper, onion, chili powder and garlic powder. Cook 3-4 minutes, stirring well, until the mushrooms start to soften and the onion browns. Turn the heat off. Add the lemon zest and juice, and toss.

Set out two plates and place 2 cups of the spinach on each. Divide the chicken with the sauce over the spinach and serve immediately.

CHICKEN MARSALA

Yield: 4 Servings (1 serving is 2 ½ cups)

Chicken Marsala gets its flavor from piling on the mushrooms and sweet Marsala wine. This recipe has loads of detoxifying mushroom but replaces the wine with balsamic vinegar for extra zip.

Ingredients

4 skinless, boneless chicken cutlets
1 teaspoon dried oregano
¼ teaspoon salt
¼ teaspoon freshly ground black pepper
2 tablespoons coconut oil
2 cloves garlic, minced
2 tablespoons unsalted butter, preferably grass-fed
½ red or yellow onion, sliced thinly (about ½ cup)
1 small zucchini thinly sliced
8 ounces white button mushrooms, sliced
1 tablespoon balsamic vinegar mixed with ⅓ cup water
¼ cup fresh basil, thinly sliced
¼ teaspoon ground flax or coconut flour

Instructions

Heat the oil over medium-high in a large skillet. Sprinkle the chicken with the oregano, salt and pepper. Add the coconut oil to the skillet along with the chicken and garlic. Cook until lightly browned (about 2-3 minutes) turning once.

Add the butter along with the onion, zucchini and mushrooms. Cook 2-3 minutes until the vegetables are soft and sprinkle with the ground flax or coconut flour. Stir well and add the balsamic water mixture. Cook 1 minute more until the sauce thickens slightly. Sprinkle with the basil. Serve immediately.

DIJON SALMON STEAKS

Yield: 4 Servings

Salmon is an excellent source of omega-3 fatty acids, which when consumed regularly can aid with cardiovascular, joint, brain and even eye health. Be sure to purchase wild salmon when available, as this will ensure the intake of far less contaminants.

Ingredients

4 6-ounce salmon steaks
1 lemon, halved
Salt and freshly ground pepper, to taste

2 tablespoons Dijon mustard
4 teaspoons fresh dill, minced

Instructions

Preheat the broiler. Lightly oil a broiler rack with high-heat cooking spray and set aside. Squeeze the lemon halves evenly over the salmon to coat with juice and set aside to rest for 5 minutes. Season the salmon steaks to taste with salt and pepper and arrange them on the broiler rack. Broil for about 4 minutes and remove the broiling pan.

Flip the steaks and spread equal amounts of the mustard over the tops. Return to the broiler and cook until salmon is just opaque, about 3-4 minutes longer. Transfer the steaks to a platter and sprinkle the dill over the top to serve.

EASY ROASTED HERB CHICKEN

Yield: 4 Servings

Roast chicken is comforting but roasting a whole bird can take some time. This version uses bone-in chicken breasts (with the skin on), so the meat is still moist and juicy, while cutting the cooking time by 1 hour.

Ingredients

4 cups broccoli florets or bok choy, chopped
2 tablespoons unsalted butter, preferably grass-fed
2 tablespoons fresh basil, chopped
2 tablespoons fresh parsley or cilantro, chopped

1 tablespoon fresh rosemary, chopped
¼ teaspoon salt
4 skin-on, bone-in chicken breasts

Instructions

Preheat the oven to 400°F. Cover a baking sheet with aluminum foil. Arrange the broccoli or the bok choy in the center of the tray. Place the chicken on top.

Place the butter, basil, rosemary, parsley or cilantro, and salt in a small bowl. Mash the herbs into the butter. Spread the butter evenly over the chicken with a spatula. Roast 25-30 minutes or until the chicken is cooked through to the bone, no longer pink, and juices run clear when pricked. Serve immediately.

FLAVORFUL FLANK STEAK

Yield: 4 Servings

Enjoy this flank steak with a large side of vegetables for a hearty dinner. Use leftovers as a protein layer on tomorrow's salad!

Ingredients

2 teaspoons paprika
1 teaspoon garlic powder
1 teaspoon onion powder
½ teaspoon dried oregano
½ teaspoon dried thyme
1 teaspoon salt
½ teaspoon freshly ground black pepper
½ teaspoon cayenne pepper
1 1-1.5-pound top round or flank steak
Unsalted butter, preferably grass-fed

Instructions

For the rub, combine paprika, garlic powder, onion powder, oregano, thyme, salt, pepper and cayenne pepper in a small bowl and mix.

Lightly coat the steak with a little grass-fed butter and sprinkle with the rub, distributing with your hands if necessary. Allow the meat to rest for 15-30 minutes at room temperature before cooking.

Grill the steak over medium-high heat for 8-10 minutes, flipping once, for medium rare. To cook on the stovetop, use a grill pan over high heat. Cook steak for 5-7 minutes, flipping once, or until it reaches desired doneness.

Slice thinly against the grain to serve.

GRILLED CHICKEN BREASTS IN TOMATO SAUCE

Yield: 4 Servings

A rich tomato sauce over chicken breasts will help you to feel fully nourished on a cold winter's night.

Ingredients

2 ripe tomatoes, halved
1 large red bell pepper, seeded and quartered
½ cup sundried tomato strips in oil, well drained
Small handful of fresh basil leaves
1 large clove garlic, crushed
1 teaspoon dried oregano
¼ teaspoon and a sprinkling of salt and freshly ground pepper
3 tablespoons coconut oil, melted
6-8 bone-in chicken breasts

Instructions

Preheat grill to high.

In a food processor, combine the tomatoes, pepper, sundried tomato strips, basil, garlic, oregano, salt and pepper. Drizzle the oil over top. Pulse a few times to break up the larger pieces, then process steadily, scraping down the sides as necessary, until the mixture forms a sauce that is mostly smooth. If the mixture is too thick, drizzle in a little more melted oil, one teaspoon at a time, until you reach the desired consistency. Taste the sauce and adjust seasoning if necessary. Set aside.

Season chicken breasts lightly with salt and pepper. Place the chicken on the hottest part of the grill and leave undisturbed for 4-5 minutes until it is opaque. Flip and cook for another 4-5 minutes until just cooked through. Allow the chicken to rest for a couple of minutes before serving. Top with sauce to taste and serve.

GRILLED LAMB CHOPS

Yield: 4 Servings

By using a variety of herbs you can upgrade grilled lamb chops into an elegant yet easy-to-serve dish that the entire family will appreciate. Be on the lookout for lamb from Australia as this will likely ensure that it is a grass-fed product.

Ingredients

¼ cup tamari (gluten-free)
 3 tablespoons olive oil
Juice of 1 lemon
3 cloves garlic, minced
⅓ cup fresh mint leaves, chopped
¼ cup fresh rosemary leaves, chopped
3 tablespoons fresh thyme leaves, chopped
¾ teaspoon freshly ground pepper
½ teaspoon salt
4 lamb chops

Instructions

In a shallow glass storage container, whisk together the tamari, oil and lemon juice. Add garlic, mint, rosemary, thyme, pepper and salt. Mix thoroughly.

Lay lamb chops in a single layer in the dish and flip a few times to coat with the herbs and marinade.

Cover and marinate for 30 minutes, flipping a few times.

Grill chops over medium heat for about for 6-7 minutes, flip, and grill for 4-5 minutes more for medium rare, or to desired doneness.

HERBED LAMB KEBABS WITH GRILLED ZUCCHINI

Yield: 4 Servings

Grab some skewers and thread this herbed lamb (or meat of your choice) for easy grilling.

Ingredients

¼ cup olive oil, plus 2 teaspoons, divided
1 large lemon, juice and zest
2 tablespoons tamari (gluten-free)
4 cloves garlic, crushed
⅓ cup chopped fresh mint
¼ cup fresh rosemary, crushed
3 tablespoons fresh thyme
½ teaspoon each salt and cracked black pepper
1½ pounds lean lamb, cut into 1-inch cubes
2 medium zucchini, sliced lengthwise, ½-inch thick
Salt and fresh ground pepper, to taste

Instructions

In a small bowl combine ¼ cup of the olive oil, lemon juice and zest and tamari and whisk to combine. Add the garlic, mint, rosemary, thyme, salt and pepper and mix well.

Spread the lamb cubes out in a glass storage dish and pour marinade over all, turning to coat all sides. Marinate the meat from 3 hours to overnight, turning pieces occasionally.

Combine the zucchini, remaining 2 teaspoons olive oil, salt and pepper in a large bowl and toss to evenly coat.

Preheat grill to medium-low. Place the meat loosely on four metal skewers, removing as much of the marinade as possible. Lay the skewers and the prepared zucchini strips on the grill and cook to desired doneness, about 6-9 minutes, turning occasionally.

MINI MEATBALL MINESTRONE SOUP

Yield: 8 Servings

Mini meatballs take the place of pasta or beans in this twist on classic minestrone. Grass-fed ground beef is rich in omega-3s and has a deep beefy flavor compared to corn-fed beef. If you shop for ground beef by the pound, freeze the extra ½ pound to make this soup another time.

Ingredients

Mini meatballs
1 pound lean ground beef
4 mushrooms, grated or chopped
2 tablespoons ground flax
¼ cup fresh basil, chopped
1 egg
¼ teaspoon salt
¼ teaspoon freshly ground black pepper
2 tablespoons coconut oil

Soup
½ yellow or red onion, chopped
2 garlic cloves, minced
1 15-ounce can diced tomatoes
1 teaspoon dried oregano
2 cups broccoli, cut into florets
2 cups cauliflower, cut into florets
32 ounces chicken or vegetable broth, low-sodium

¼ cup lemon juice (from 1 lemon)

Instructions

Prepare the meatballs. Place the beef, mushrooms, ground flax, basil, egg, salt and pepper in a large bowl. Mix well. Form into 1-inch meatballs and transfer to a plate.

Heat a large stockpot over medium heat and add the coconut oil. Add the meatballs and cook 2-3 minutes, turning occasionally until the meatballs brown. Scatter the onions and garlic around the meatballs. Add the diced tomatoes and oregano and cook 1-2 minutes, gently stirring until the onions soften. Add the broccoli, cauliflower and broth. Bring to a simmer over medium heat and cook 5-6 minutes, until the broccoli is tender. Before serving, stir in the lemon juice.

MOUTHWATERING MEATLOAF

Yield: 4 Servings

Meatloaf is an American classic, and is usually made with breadcrumbs. In this version, juicy, grated zucchini takes the place of bread, keeping the loaf moist with fewer calories and smarter carbs.

Ingredients

1 tablespoon olive oil
½ yellow or red onion, finely chopped
3 garlic cloves, minced
1 teaspoon chili powder, mild or hot
½ teaspoon dried oregano
¼ teaspoon freshly ground black pepper
⅛ teaspoon cinnamon (optional)
2 tablespoons tamari (gluten-free) or ½ teaspoon salt
1 cup zucchini, grated (about 1 small zucchini)
1 pound lean ground beef
1 egg
1 tablespoon tomato paste mixed with 1 teaspoon coconut oil
⅓ cup ground flaxseed (optional—this will help bind the meatloaf)

Instructions

Preheat the oven to 400°F. Heat a large skillet over medium-high heat and add the olive oil. Add the onions, garlic, chili powder, oregano, salt, black pepper and cinnamon, if using. Cook 3-4 minutes, stirring often, until the vegetables soften and begin to brown. Stir in the tamari or salt. Transfer to a large bowl and cool slightly about 5 minutes.

Add the zucchini and toss. Add the beef, egg and optional flax. Mix well. Transfer to a baking dish and cover with the tomato paste and olive oil mixture. Bake 45-50 minutes until the meatloaf is firm around the edges and cooked through. Rest for 5 minutes before serving.

PALEO FAJITAS

Yield: Serves 4

Festive fajitas make for a fast and satisfying meal. Turn leftover steak from another recipe into a quick-to-make version of this meal (warm meat for 5 minutes in a 350°F preheated oven).

Ingredients

1¼ pounds flank steak
1 tablespoon coconut oil
2 teaspoons chili powder
½ teaspoon cumin
½ teaspoon dried oregano
¼ teaspoon salt
¼ teaspoon freshly ground pepper
2 cups Grilled Peppers and Onions (see Vegetable Sides)
1 head butter or Boston bib lettuce
2 limes, cut into wedges

Instructions

Rub the steak with the coconut oil. Sprinkle the meat with chili powder, cumin, oregano, salt and pepper. Heat a large skillet or grill over medium heat. Transfer the flank steak to the skillet or grill and cook 8-10 minutes (or less if a thinner cut of meat), turning occasionally until the meat is pink in the center but not translucent. Rest steak 5 minutes on a cutting board and thinly slice against the grain.

Break the lettuce head into separate leaves and place 2 slices of the meat along with a spoonful of the peppers and onions. Repeat with remaining leaves and meat. Serve with lime wedges.

RAINBOW STUFFED PEPPERS

Yield: 4 Servings

Homey stuffed peppers are the perfect cold-weather comfort food.

Ingredients

4 red, yellow or orange bell peppers
½ pound lean ground turkey
2 stalks celery, grated
2 cups mushrooms, grated
½ cup parsley, chopped
4 garlic cloves, minced
1 egg
2 tablespoon ground flax
¼ teaspoon salt
¼ teaspoon freshly ground black pepper
1 slice uncooked bacon, chopped
2 tablespoons tomato paste
2 cups chicken broth, low-sodium

Instructions

Cut the tops of the peppers and clean out the seeds. Place the turkey, celery, mushrooms, parsley, garlic, egg, flax, salt and pepper in a large bowl. Mix well.

Place the bacon in a large stockpot over medium heat. Cook 4-5 minutes, until the bacon crisps and releases its fat. Set the peppers in the stockpot, cut side up, on top of the bacon. Divide the turkey mixture between the four peppers, filling with a spoon.

Tuck the tomato paste into a corner of the pot, around the peppers. Pour in the chicken broth around the peppers. Increase the heat to medium, and bring to a simmer. Cover and cook 35-40 minutes, until the peppers are soft and the filling is cooked through. Serve immediately.

SAVORY STEAK WITH MUSHROOMS

Yield: 4 Servings

Grass-fed steak is full of flavor, but when paired with mushrooms, shallots and oil you have the ideal combination. Enjoy this recipe for a special meal at home with your loved ones.

Ingredients

1-1½-pound sirloin steak (1-inch thickness)
½ teaspoon salt plus 1 pinch
½ teaspoon freshly ground pepper
1 tablespoon coconut oil
2 teaspoons butter, preferably grass-fed
2 shallots, chopped
8 ounces sliced mushrooms (button, cremini, shitake all work well)
1 tablespoon fresh thyme, minced (or ¾ teaspoon dried)
6 cups baby arugula, spinach or other chopped tender greens

Dressing
2 tablespoons olive oil
1 tablespoon red wine vinegar
1 teaspoon Dijon mustard
1 teaspoon lemon zest (optional)
Salt and freshly ground pepper to taste

Instructions

Preheat broiler and lightly oil broiler pan. Set aside. Pat steak dry with paper towel, and season lightly with salt and pepper on both sides. Broil steak 3-4 inches from heating element for 4-5 minutes and turn. Broil for 4-5 minutes more for medium-rare.

Remove from heat and tent with foil while preparing the mushrooms. Heat coconut oil and butter in large sauté pan over medium heat.

Add shallots, mushrooms and a pinch of salt, and sauté 3-5 minutes until mushrooms are just tender. Stir in thyme and sauté until mushrooms reach desired tenderness. Remove from heat.

While mushrooms are sautéing, in a small bowl, whisk together oil, red wine vinegar, mustard, lemon zest, if using, and salt and pepper. Slice the steak into thick strips.

On a serving platter or individual plates, make a layer of lettuce, add the warm mushroom and shallot mixture, dress lightly, and top with steak strips.

SLOW-COOKER COCONUT SALMON

Yield: 4 Servings

If cooking fish seems daunting, then this no- fuss, slow-cooker recipe is perfect for you. Using a slow cooker ensures that the fish isn't overcooked while creating an over-the-top, deeply flavored sauce infused with garlic and chili. If you're not a fan of heat, omit the chili flakes and use mild chili powder.

Ingredients

½ cup unsweetened coconut milk (from carton, not canned)
2 scallions, thinly sliced
4 cloves garlic, minced
2 tablespoons coconut oil
½ teaspoon salt
1 teaspoon chili powder, mild or hot
¼ teaspoon crushed red chili flakes (optional)
4 4-ounce salmon filets, skin removed
2 tablespoons fresh cilantro or parsley, minced
4 cups baby spinach

Instructions

Place the coconut milk, scallions, garlic, coconut oil, salt, chili powder and red chili flakes in the slow cooker, and stir well. Add the salmon filets and turn them to coat in the coconut mixture. Set the slow cooker to low and cook 2 hours, until the salmon is cooked through but still tender. During the last 20 minutes of cooking, layer the cilantro or parsley and spinach on top. Serve immediately.

SLOW-COOKER PORK LOIN WITH MUSTARD AND ROSEMARY

Yield: Serves 6

A slow-cooker pork roast never comes out dry when you set your cooker to low and follow the simple timing guidelines. Note: These roasts don't come in small sizes—they usually start at around 2½-3 pounds—but you can use the extra meat for salads and other dishes.

Ingredients

2 tablespoons Dijon mustard
2 tablespoon fresh rosemary, chopped

4 garlic cloves, thinly sliced
1 3-pound end pork loin roast

Instructions

Place one tablespoon of the mustard inside the slow cooker. Add the pork and spread the remaining tablespoon of mustard over the pork. Sprinkle the rosemary and garlic on top and cover.

Set the slow cooker to low and cook 3 -3½ hours until the pork roast is cooked through but still slightly pink in the center. Transfer the roast to a cutting board and rest 5 minutes before slicing.

SLOW-COOKER SHRIMP DIAVOLO

Yield: 4 Servings

Diavolo—"devil" in Italian—is a sinfully delicious spicy tomato sauce. If you are not a fan of heat, simply leave out the chili flakes or replace them with 2 tablespoons chopped fresh basil or ¼ teaspoon dried oregano.

Ingredients

1 pound medium shrimp, shelled, tails removed
1 bunch asparagus, trimmed and cut on the bias
1 cup diced canned tomatoes

1 tablespoon tomato paste
1 teaspoon red chili flakes
¼ cup parsley, chopped

Instructions

Place shrimp, asparagus, canned tomatoes, tomato paste, and chili flakes in the slow cooker on low heat. Toss well and cook 1½ hours until the shrimp is tender. Sprinkle with parsley and serve immediately.

SOLE FILET OVER GREENS

Yield: 4 Servings

The sweetness from the blueberries will balance this fish dish and provide you with an assortment of antioxidants for great body composition and overall good health.

Ingredients

1 tablespoon coconut oil
2 large shallots, sliced
4 4-ounce sole fillets, skin removed
½ teaspoon each salt and freshly ground pepper
½ pint blueberries
6 ounces baby spinach, arugula or a combination

Instructions

Melt the coconut oil in a large skillet or Dutch oven over medium heat. Add the shallot and sauté for 2-3 minutes until soft. Remove from skillet and set aside.

Reduce the heat to medium-low and transfer the sole fillets to the pan. Sprinkle with half of the salt and pepper. Cook for about 4 minutes, gently flip, sprinkle with remaining salt and pepper, and cook on second side for 4-5 minutes or until the fish flakes easily with a fork.

Transfer fillets to a platter and set aside in a warm oven. Add the blueberries, baby greens and shallots and cover pan for 1 minute. Remove cover and stir gently, cooking for about 2 more minutes or until hot and greens are wilted.

Make 4 beds of the wilted greens and blueberries and top each bed with 1 sole fillet to serve.

TURKEY CHILI

Yield: 3 Servings

Fresh cilantro and lime give this standard chili pizzazz. It stores well in the refrigerator for five days, or it can be frozen in two-cup portions. Leftovers are perfect for a no-hassle lunch at the office.

Ingredients

2 tablespoons coconut oil
1 pound ground lean white meat turkey
½ cup fresh cilantro, chopped
½ yellow or red onion, finely chopped
3 garlic cloves, minced
2 tablespoons chili powder, mild or hot
2 teaspoons ground cumin
1 teaspoon dried oregano
6 tablespoons canned tomato paste
1 32-ounce container chicken broth, low-sodium
1 15-ounce canned diced tomatoes
1 small zucchini, sliced
1 cup kale, stemmed and chopped or torn into bite-sized pieces
¼ cup fresh lime juice (about 2 limes)

Instructions

Heat a large stockpot over medium heat. Add the coconut oil. Add the turkey meat and sear 1-2 minutes without stirring. Scatter the cilantro, onion and garlic around the turkey meat and cook 2-3 minutes more, stirring once or twice to break up the meat. Add the chili powder, cumin, and oregano and stir. Add the tomato paste and cook 1 minute more, stirring once or twice until the paste becomes fragrant.

Add the chicken broth, the diced tomatoes, zucchini and kale and bring to a simmer over medium heat for 20-30 minutes until the meat is cooked through and the vegetables are tender. Add the lime juice and serve immediately.

QUICK INDIAN TURKEY BURGER SALAD

Yield: 4 Servings

Indian spices are used to create this flavorful turkey burger. Prepare the patties and sauce ahead of time so you can come home to a quick-and-easy meal.

Ingredients

1 egg
1 pound lean ground turkey
2 tablespoons ground flaxseed
¼ cup chopped scallions
1 tablespoon Dijon mustard
1 clove garlic, minced

1 tablespoon minced ginger
1 teaspoon curry powder
½ teaspoon cumin
¾ teaspoon salt
½ teaspoon pepper

Sauce

½ cup homemade mayonnaise
½ teaspoon curry powder
2 tablespoons minced fresh cilantro

1 teaspoon lemon juice
2 drops NuNaturals vanilla stevia (optional)

Mayonnaise

1 whole egg
½ teaspoon of Dijon mustard or 1 teaspoon dry mustard powder

2 tablespoons lemon juice
¼ teaspoon salt
1 cup light olive oil

Salad

4 cups sliced red leaf lettuce
1 tomato, chopped

2 cups sprouts (broccoli, pea or alfalfa)

Instructions

Preheat grill or grill pan to medium heat.

In a large bowl, add the egg and whisk until lightly beaten. Add the turkey, flaxseed, scallions, mustard, garlic, ginger, curry, salt and pepper, and mix gently with your hands. Form 4 equal patties.

Spray the grill or grill pan with high-heat cooking oil and cook burgers until cooked through, 5-6 minutes per side (165°F).

While the burgers are cooking, prepare the mayonnaise for the sauce. Add all mayonnaise ingredients to a wide mouth Mason jar. Let the oil rise to the top. Place immersion blender at the very bottom of the jar and blend. As the mayo emulsifies, slowly tilt the immersion blender to allow the remaining oil to blend. Refrigerate any unused portion in an airtight container and use within two weeks. Prepare the sauce. In a small bowl combine the mayonnaise, curry powder, cilantro, lemon juice and stevia.Make 4 salad beds with equal portions of the lettuce, tomato and sprouts.

Top with a burger and dress with sauce, to taste.

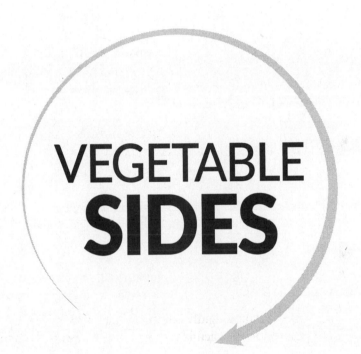

VEGETABLE
SIDES

BROCCOLI ALMONDINE

Yield: 2 Servings

Crunchy almonds add interest and a good quality fat to this fast, healthy side dish. If you can't find slivered almonds in your local supermarket, you can chop the nuts with a knife or in a mini-chopper.

Ingredients

1 tablespoon coconut oil
1 bunch broccoli, cut into florets (about 4 cups)
1 teaspoon chili powder, mild or hot

¼ teaspoon salt
1 lemon, zest and juice
¼ cup almonds, slivered or chopped

Instructions

Heat a large skillet over medium-high heat. Add the coconut oil, broccoli, chili powder, salt and lemon zest.

Cook 1-2 minutes, until the broccoli browns slightly.

Cover and reduce the heat to low and cook another 2 minutes, until the broccoli is tender. Add the lemon juice and almonds. Toss well. Serve immediately.

CLASSIC VEGGIE STIR-FRY

Yield: 2 Servings

Takeout fans will warm to this fast stir-fry that you can cook in less than 5 minutes. To cut back on prep time, use a food processor to chop the onions and garlic and buy pre-cut broccoli from the produce aisle.

Ingredients

1 tablespoon coconut oil
1 red or yellow onion, chopped
1 green bell pepper, seeded, chopped
5 ounces mushrooms, quartered
2 cups broccoli, cut in florets

2 cloves garlic, minced
4 teaspoons fresh ginger, minced
Pinch of turmeric (optional)
1 tablespoon tamari (gluten-free)

Instructions

Heat a large skillet over medium high-heat. Add the coconut oil, onion, pepper, mushrooms, broccoli, garlic, ginger and turmeric, if using, and cook 3-4 minutes, stirring often until the vegetables soften and begin to brown.

Turn the heat off and add the turmeric and tamari along with 2 tablespoons of water. Toss well. Serve immediately.

DIJON ASPARAGUS

Yield: 2 Servings

Tangy Dijon mustard makes a tasty glaze for this cleansing spring vegetable that you can find year-round in your local grocery store. When shopping for asparagus, look for spears with firm tips that aren't mushy. The stalks should be firm and unwrinkled.

Ingredients

1 tablespoon coconut oil
1 pound asparagus, trimmed, cut into 1-inch pieces
1 tablespoon Dijon mustard
2 garlic cloves, minced
½ teaspoon stevia

Instructions

Heat a large skillet over medium heat and add the coconut oil. Add the asparagus and cook 1-2 minutes, stirring often, until the asparagus begins to brown.

Reduce the heat to low and add the mustard, garlic, stevia and 2 tablespoons of water. Cover and cook 1 minute until the asparagus is tender. Serve immediately.

GARLIC BROCCOLI

Yield: 2 Servings

Garlic lovers will enjoy this savory yet light garlicky broccoli side dish. There's no need to steam the broccoli first—covering allows the natural water content to cook the broccoli through.

Ingredients

1 tablespoon coconut oil
4 cups broccoli, cut into florets
4 garlic cloves, minced
¼ teaspoon salt
¼ teaspoon crushed red pepper flakes

Instructions

Heat a large skillet over medium-high heat. Add the coconut oil, broccoli, garlic, salt and red pepper flakes. Cook 2 minutes, stirring often until the garlic becomes fragrant. Reduce the heat to low and cover.

Cook 2-3 minutes until the broccoli is tender and cooked through. Serve immediately.

GINGERED BOK CHOY

Yield: 2 Servings

Bok choy is a delicious Asian cruciferous vegetable, in the same family as kale and broccoli. If your local market doesn't carry bok choy, you can also substitute the same amount of kale or broccoli. Just slice kale or cut broccoli into florets before cooking.

Ingredients

1 teaspoon coconut oil
4 teaspoons fresh ginger, mined
4 garlic cloves, minced
1 pound bok choy, chopped
¼ teaspoon salt
1 tablespoon butter, preferably grass-fed
1 lime, zested and juiced

Instructions

Heat a large stockpot over medium-high heat. Add the coconut oil, ginger and garlic, and cook about 1 minute until fragrant. Add the bok choy and salt, cook 2-3 minutes more, stirring often. Add the butter, lime zest and juice. Toss well. Serve immediately.

GRILLED PEPPERS AND ONIONS

Yield: 2 Servings

If you're a fan of grilled peppers and onions on a sausage sandwich, then you'll love this side dish. Leftovers are ideal in scrambled eggs or served next to pork or beef, gently warmed.

Ingredients

1 tablespoon coconut oil
2 onions, peeled, sliced
2 red, orange, or yellow bell peppers, seeded, and sliced
½ teaspoon salt
Pinch of turmeric (optional)
1 teaspoon fresh rosemary leaves, chopped

Instructions

Heat a large skillet over medium-high heat. Add the coconut oil. Add the onions, peppers, salt, turmeric, if using, and rosemary. Cook 3-4 minutes, stirring often, until the peppers and onions soften. Serve immediately.

LEMONY ASPARAGUS

Yield: 2 Servings

Lemon and asparagus have "spring-fling flavor" in this zesty recipe that is fancy enough for evening entertaining. Short on time during the week? Trim and slice asparagus, and zest and juice the lemon in advance. Store both in the fridge for up to 24 hours.

Ingredients

1 tablespoon coconut oil
1 pound asparagus, trimmed, cut into 1-inch pieces
2 lemons, zested and juiced (use less lemon, if you prefer)
¼ cup fresh basil leaves, sliced

Instructions

Heat a large skillet over medium-high heat. Add the coconut oil, asparagus and lemon zest. Toss well and cook 2-3 minutes until the asparagus starts to soften.

Reduce the heat to low and cover. Cook an additional 2-3 minutes until the asparagus is tender. Add the lemon juice. Cook 1 minute more, uncovered, to allow the lemon juice to reduce. Add the basil and toss. Serve immediately.

SESAME SPINACH

Yield: 2 Servings

Sesame and tamari make a perfect match for this superfood rich in a multitude of nutrients, including folate, fiber and vitamin A. Serve this along with salmon or grilled beef for a satisfying meal.

Ingredients

1 tablespoon coconut oil
1 pound baby spinach
1 tablespoon tamari (gluten-free)
1 tablespoon sesame seeds

Instructions

Heat a large stockpot over high heat and add the coconut oil. Add the spinach and press down with a small lid until all the spinach has wilted, 1-2 minutes.

Turn the heat to low, and add the tamari and sesame seeds. Toss well to coat. Serve immediately.

ZUCCHINI AND SPINACH WITH BROWN BUTTER

Yield: 2 Servings

Browning butter gives this dish a wonderful nutty taste that dresses up the plain vegetables. Fresh sage leaves become mild and crispy when cooked with butter and add an additional punch of flavor.

Ingredients

1 tablespoons unsalted butter, preferably grass-fed
½ teaspoon sage or 4-6 fresh sage leaves, chopped (optional)
1 small zucchini, thinly sliced
5 ounces baby spinach
¼ teaspoon salt

Instructions

Place the butter in a large skillet over medium heat. If using sage, add the sage and cook 30 seconds. For fresh sage, cook until the leaves crisp. Add the zucchini, baby spinach and a sprinkle of the salt. Toss well. Serve immediately.

APPENDIX:
WEEKLY
SHOPPING LISTS

NOTE ON SHOPPING LISTS

For your convenience, we have included shopping lists for each week's meal plan. You should use these as guidelines for what to buy each week. As sizes, amounts and types of foods vary, it's impossible to make a shopping list that works for every person. We have attempted to create shopping lists that build from one week to the next, so you don't find your cupboards becoming overloaded with multiple versions of the same items. Before you go shopping, please check your pantry, fridge and freezer and cross off any items you may not need. Also, if there is a recipe you don't plan to make, or if you are considering substitutes in recipes, make sure to make notes before you go to the grocery store.

Also remember that most of the recipes in this book yield four servings. The shopping lists were designed to go hand-in-hand with the recipes and meal plans. If you are cooking for one or two and cutting recipes in half, you should also cut the amount of groceries you buy in half.

SHOPPING LIST: WEEK 1

PROTEIN

- ☐ 1 container of protein powder
- ☐ 1 3-pound end pork loin roast
- ☐ 4 cups cubed chicken, cooked
- ☐ 8 chicken breasts
- ☐ 1 dozen eggs
- ☐ 6 ounces sliced gluten-free deli meat of your choice (e.g., roast beef, chicken, turkey, etc.)
- ☐ Protein of your choice (chicken, turkey, lean steak, etc.) for "Roll Your Own" Salad
- ☐ 1¼ pounds flank steak
- ☐ 12 ounces cooked turkey breast
- ☐ 1 pound ground lean white meat turkey
- ☐ 1 small package of bacon
- ☐ 4 4-ounce salmon filets
- ☐ 4 5-ounce cans chunk light tuna packed in extra virgin olive oil, well drained

FRUITS & VEGETABLES

- ☐ 1 medium sweet potato
- ☐ 1 butternut squash
- ☐ 1 baked potato
- ☐ 1 shallot
- ☐ 1 pint grape tomatoes
- ☐ 1 pint cherry tomatoes
- ☐ 1 large tomato
- ☐ 1 small package of carrots
- ☐ 1 5-ounce package mushrooms
- ☐ 4 red bell pepper
- ☐ 2 red, orange, or yellow bell peppers
- ☐ 1 package broccoli slaw (or other shredded veggies of choices)
- ☐ 1 head cauliflower
- ☐ 4 heads broccoli
- ☐ 4 avocados
- ☐ 2 cucumbers
- ☐ 2 red onions
- ☐ 5 yellow onions
- ☐ 1 bunch scallions
- ☐ 3 large containers baby spinach
- ☐ 1 container salad greens of your choice
- ☐ 1 head butter or Boston bib lettuce
- ☐ 5 large heads of romaine lettuce
- ☐ 1 large container of mesclun greens
- ☐ 1 head of collard greens
- ☐ 1 pound of bok choy
- ☐ 1 head kale
- ☐ 2 pounds asparagus
- ☐ 3 cups green beans
- ☐ 1 container bean sprouts
- ☐ 7 limes
- ☐ 5 lemons
- ☐ 1 small zucchini
- ☐ 1 bunch of leeks
- ☐ 2 apples
- ☐ 1 bag frozen low-glycemic fruit (for "Roll Your Own" Shakes)
- ☐ 1 bag of frozen raspberries
- ☐ 1 bag frozen peaches

HERBS & SPICES

☐ 1 container fresh rosemary
☐ 2 containers fresh basil leaves
☐ 1 container fresh parsley
☐ 1 container fresh mint leaves
☐ 1 container fresh cilantro
☐ 4 bulbs garlic
☐ 1 sea salt shaker
☐ 1 ground pepper grinder
☐ 1 jar dried oregano
☐ 1 jar garlic powder

☐ 1 jar chili powder
☐ 1 jar cumin
☐ 1 jar dried basil
☐ 1 jar crushed red pepper flakes
☐ 1 large piece of ginger
☐ 1 jar nutmeg
☐ 1 jar orange zest
☐ 1 jar turmeric (optional)
☐ 1 jar vanilla extract

PANTRY ITEMS

☐ 1 can black beans
☐ 1 package of brown rice
☐ 1 jar of Dijon mustard
☐ 1 jar roasted peppers
☐ 1 small bottle red wine vinegar
☐ 1 bottle extra-virgin olive oil
☐ 1 box of green tea
☐ 1 large bag of chia seeds
☐ 1 container of stevia (optional)
☐ 1 15-ounce jar artichoke hearts in water, drained
☐ 1 jar pitted green olives
☐ 1 jar pitted black olives
☐ 1 stick of butter, preferably grass-fed
☐ 1 small bag of pine nuts
☐ 1 bag of unsalted almonds
☐ 1 small bag walnuts

☐ ½ teaspoon cinnamon
☐ 1 bottle coconut oil
☐ 2 containers chicken broth, low-sodium
☐ 1 32-ounce container of unsweetened almond milk
☐ 1 bottle raw unpasteurized apple cider vinegar
☐ 1 16-ounce container unsweetened coconut milk
☐ 1 bag cocoa nibs (or a container of unsweetened cocoa powder)
☐ 1 small bottle flaxseed oil (optional)
☐ 1 can of tomato paste
☐ 1 15-ounce canned diced tomatoes
☐ 2 15-ounce jar artichoke hearts
☐ 1 small jar capers
☐ 1 bottle tamari (gluten-free)
☐ 1 small package sesame seeds

SHOPPING LIST: WEEK 2

METABOLIC MEALS PLAN

PROTEIN

- [ ] 1 container protein powder (if needed)
- [ ] 12 skinless, boneless chicken breasts
- [ ] 1 dozen eggs
- [ ] 1½ pound flank steak
- [ ] 1-1½ pound sirloin steak (1-inch thickness)
- [ ] 1 pound lean ground beef
- [ ] 1½ pounds lean lamb, cut into 1-inch cubes
- [ ] 1½ pound lean ground turkey
- [ ] Protein of your choice (chicken, turkey, lean steak, etc.)
- [ ] 2 7.5-ounce cans wild salmon
- [ ] 1 small package of smoked wild salmon (3 ounces)
- [ ] 2½ pounds medium shrimp, shelled and deveined
- [ ] 1 cooked turkey or chicken sausage
- [ ] Bacon, crumbled

FRUITS & VEGETABLES

- [ ] 7 red, yellow or orange bell peppers
- [ ] 1 bunch of celery
- [ ] 1 carrot
- [ ] 1 medium sweet potato
- [ ] 1 baked potato
- [ ] 1 acorn squash
- [ ] 1 bunch kale
- [ ] 2 red onions
- [ ] 3 yellow onions
- [ ] 2 shallots
- [ ] 1 bunch of scallions
- [ ] 2 8 ounces sliced mushrooms (button, cremini, shitake all work well)
- [ ] 3 limes
- [ ] 5 lemons
- [ ] 1 cup green beans
- [ ] 4 avocados
- [ ] 3 containers bean sprouts
- [ ] 1 head spinach
- [ ] 1 large container baby spinach
- [ ] 1 large head red leaf lettuce
- [ ] 3 large heads romaine lettuce
- [ ] 1 large container of mixed greens
- [ ] 1 large container arugula
- [ ] 4 heads broccoli
- [ ] 1 head cauliflower
- [ ] 4 tomatoes
- [ ] 1 container grape tomatoes
- [ ] 1 container cherry tomatoes
- [ ] 1 package snap peas
- [ ] 1 bunch asparagus
- [ ] 3 medium zucchini
- [ ] 1 bag of frozen cherries
- [ ] 1 bag of frozen low-glycemic fruit (for "Roll Your Own" shakes)

HERBS & SPICES

- ☐ 3 bulbs of garlic
- ☐ 2 bunches of fresh parsley
- ☐ 1 jar cinnamon
- ☐ 1 container fresh cilantro leaves
- ☐ 1 container fresh basil leaves
- ☐ 1 small piece of fresh ginger
- ☐ 1 jar curry powder

- ☐ 1 jar cayenne pepper
- ☐ 1 jar of dried sage
- ☐ 1 container fresh thyme
- ☐ 1 container fresh dill
- ☐ 1 container fresh mint
- ☐ 1 container fresh rosemary

PANTRY ITEMS

- ☐ 1 container unsweetened almond milk
- ☐ 1 container unsweetened coconut milk
- ☐ 2 tablespoons balsamic vinegar
- ☐ 1 small bag ground flax
- ☐ 1 small can tomato paste
- ☐ 1 can of black beans (or beans of your choice)
- ☐ 1 bag shredded unsweetened coconut
- ☐ 1 small jar sesame oil
- ☐ 1 stick of butter, preferably grass-fed
- ☐ 1 small jar of sundried tomato strips in oil
- ☐ 1 small container almond flour
- ☐ 2 containers chicken broth, low-sodium

- ☐ 1 bottle almond butter
- ☐ 1 small bag or container unsalted almonds
- ☐ 1 jar artichokes
- ☐ 1 can pitted black olives
- ☐ 1 bag of mixed nuts or seeds (e.g., walnuts, almonds, macadamia, sunflower seeds)
- ☐ 1 bottle light olive oil
- ☐ 1 bottle tahini
- ☐ 1 container green tea bags
- ☐ 2 15-ounce cans diced tomatoes
- ☐ 1 jar Kalamata olives
- ☐ 1 bag quinoa

SHOPPING LIST: WEEK 3

PROTEIN

- ☐ 1 container protein powder
- ☐ 1 dozen eggs
- ☐ 1 pound lean ground beef
- ☐ 1 1-1.5-pound top round or flank steak
- ☐ 1 24-ounce flank steak
- ☐ 4 skinless, boneless chicken cutlets
- ☐ 4 large chicken breasts, boneless, skinless
- ☐ 1¼ pounds chicken breasts
- ☐ 2 cups diced cooked white chicken

- ☐ 12 thin slices high-quality gluten-free deli roast beef
- ☐ Protein of your choice (chicken, turkey, lean steak, etc. for "Roll Your Own" salads)
- ☐ 4 6-ounce salmon steaks
- ☐ 1 can of salmon
- ☐ 4 4-ounce sole fillets, skin removed
- ☐ Bacon, crumbled
- ☐ ½ pound Italian gluten-free turkey sausage

FRUITS & VEGETABLES

- ☐ 2 large container of baby spinach
- ☐ 1 container salad greens of choice
- ☐ 1 large container mesclun greens
- ☐ 1 large head romaine lettuce
- ☐ 1 small container arugula
- ☐ 1 carrot
- ☐ 5 red or yellow onions
- ☐ 2 red onions
- ☐ 1 sweet onion
- ☐ 2 large shallots
- ☐ 1 small zucchini
- ☐ 1 8 ounce container white button mushrooms
- ☐ 1 5-ounce container of mushrooms
- ☐ 1 head raw collard greens
- ☐ 1 12-ounce bag broccoli slaw mix
- ☐ 1 butternut squash
- ☐ 3 red or orange bell pepper
- ☐ 1 green bell pepper

- ☐ 1 pound asparagus
- ☐ 1 cup green beans
- ☐ 3 heads broccoli
- ☐ 1 pound bok choy
- ☐ 1 cup bean sprouts
- ☐ 1 zucchini
- ☐ 2 pints cherry or grape tomatoes
- ☐ 1 tomato
- ☐ 1 cucumber
- ☐ 4 lemons
- ☐ 3 avocados
- ☐ 1 medium sweet potato
- ☐ 1 medium baked potato
- ☐ 1 pint blueberries
- ☐ 1 apple
- ☐ 1 bag of frozen fruit (for "Roll Your Own" shakes)

HERBS & SPICES

- ☐ 1 container fresh mint leaves
- ☐ 1 container fresh rosemary
- ☐ 2 teaspoons finely minced fresh ginger
- ☐ 2 containers fresh basil
- ☐ 1 cup basil or baby arugula
- ☐ 1 container fresh cilantro
- ☐ 1 container fresh dill
- ☐ 2 teaspoons paprika
- ☐ 1 jar dried thyme
- ☐ 1 jar onion powder
- ☐ 1 small bunch parsley
- ☐ 3 bulbs of garlic
- ☐ 1 piece of fresh ginger

PANTRY ITEMS

- ☐ 1 container unsweetened almond milk
- ☐ 1 container unsweetened coconut milk
- ☐ 2 sticks butter, preferably grass-fed
- ☐ 1 jar artichokes
- ☐ 1 can pitted black olives
- ☐ 1 container chicken broth, low-sodium
- ☐ 1 small container tomato paste
- ☐ 1 can of beans of choice (e.g., black beans)